OVARIAN CANCER

OVARIAN CANCER

DON'T LET IT KILL YOU

by Lyn Thompson

Published by Westminster Publishing Limited
PO Box 50253, London EC2P 2WZ, United Kingdom

© 2006 Westminster Publishing Limited.
All rights reserved.

www.westminsterpublishing.org

No part of this publication may be reproduced, stored in a retrieval system, or transmitted in any form or by any means, electronic, mechanical, photocopying, recording or otherwise, without either the prior permission of the publishers, or a licence permitting restricted copying in the United Kingdom issued by the Copyright Licensing Agency, 90 Tottenham Court Road, London W1T 4LP.

Lyn Thompson has asserted her moral right to be identified as the author of this work in accordance with the Copyright, Design and Patents Act 1988.

First published 2006
ISBN: 0-9546855-6-3

British Library Cataloguing in Publication Data
A catalogue record for this book is available from the British Library

Project Development Manager: Hazel Scott
Cover Designer: Julie Martin
Produced by Westminster Publishing

Printed and bound in the EU

CONTENTS

Introduction	7
1. Early beginnings	10
2. Looming close	16
3. Knocked over with a feather	22
4. Operation Kingston, Surrey that is	28
5. First hint of something wrong	33
6. Hello Queen Charlotte's	47
7. Operation and dreaded E. Coli	54
8. Home at last	67
9. First chemo	72
10. Fighting to survive	83
11. Overdosed on chemo	97
12. Losing my hair, losing my faith	105
13. At last, final chemo	114
14. Awareness is vital	118
15. It's back	123
16. Vincey	125
Ovacome	126
Ovarian Cancer Action	127

Thank You

Vincey. My love. My soul mate. My friend. My husband. The two small words "thank you" cannot describe adequately my debt of gratitude to you. They do not seem big enough for the care and devotion you bestowed on me. I would not have got through it without you. Thank you, my love.

Jacqueline. My wonderful daughter. Always there, always supportive, no matter what the circumstances.

Natalia, Alexandra and Nicolas. My three beautiful grandchildren. Thank you for all your moments of entertainment and for making me laugh when I felt like crying.

My sisters Pauline and Frances, my brother Pierce and my brother-in-law Joe. I could not have asked for more. Your support was unstinting and given so unselfishly.

My many nieces, nephews and my two sisters-in-laws. Thank you for caring.

Norma, a dear old friend. Thank you for being such a good friend over the years and for keeping my head straight as the editor of this book.

Rosemary. Thank you for your friendship.

Friends, work colleagues and neighbours. Theo, Richard and Marcelle, Sandy, Sabrina, Syed, Tim, the two Toms, Betty, Nesta and all the others too numerous to mention. Thank you.

INTRODUCTION

The trouble with ovarian cancer is that you don't know you have it until it is almost too late and by then, you are asking yourself how long you have to live.

Known as the silent killer, it is one of the most difficult cancers to identify. The symptoms are so ordinary that most women dismiss them as everyday aches and pains, not realising the danger they are in.

The vast majority of women are not diagnosed until they are at stage three, a stage the medical profession describes as challenging. In plain English this means that you have little chance of survival.

And of all the women diagnosed at this stage, seventy-five per cent will be dead within two years. The survival rate is dire, but what is even more heart-rending is that many of the deaths could be avoided.

Deaths could be reduced dramatically if women were more clued-up about the symptoms. Unlike the well-publicised symptoms of breast cancer, there are no lumps and bumps to help with identification. Nor is there a screening programme. You are on your own and your best chance of success is early diagnosis. But to achieve that, you need to be aware of the changes taking place in your body.

When I was diagnosed with ovarian cancer in May 2004, I was woefully ignorant of the disease and failed miserably to recognise the signs. Like most women, I had heard of it, but that was the sum total of my knowledge. I did not know that in the UK, it killed over one hundred women a week. I did not know that the majority of women were diagnosed at such an advanced stage that they have little chance of survival. And I did not know how I could have gone through life and been so unaware, so ignorant of these bleak facts. It's not as if I am a stranger to cancer. I have already had it twice before - bladder cancer ten years ago and breast cancer four years ago.

But nothing prepared me for this one. My usually laid-back attitude to cancer was shattered as I realised the terrible significance of what lay ahead for both my family and me.

The certainties in my life that had always been my mainstay disappeared in a puff of smoke. I now had to come to terms with a cancer that was alien to me, one that made demands on my body that I could barely conceive and which I did not even want to think about.

It turned my world upside down and in the process nearly took my life twice. The first time was from the killer bug, E.coli, which I picked up in hospital after I had a hysterectomy to try to remove the cancer. I lay in Queen Charlotte's Hospital in Hammersmith for nearly three weeks, hardly able to move and wondering daily whether I was going to live or die.

But if I thought that was the worst of it, I was in for a rude awakening. Still weak from the effects of E.coli, my next encounter with death was two large overdoses of chemotherapy. The drug, which is a deadly poison, wrecked my body and I became so frail that I was in danger of vanishing altogether. Not surprisingly, I was fast coming to the conclusion that the cure was more dangerous than the disease.

Yet despite the setbacks, I promised myself that if I survived I would write a book alerting women to the danger they were in unless they took control of their bodies. Every harrowing detail of my close encounters with three lots of cancer would be included. My blasé attitude to it, my ignorance of the symptoms of ovarian cancer, my fight to survive bugs and overdoses and finally my battle to bring normality back to my life as I tried to reduce the hurt that was ripping my family apart.

I was determined to write a book that would be a wake up call for women everywhere. I wanted to make women more aware of their bodies and to check for symptoms regularly - they are all listed at the back of this book.

But what I wished for more than anything else was to reduce the number of women dying unnecessarily. A first small step in improving early detection rates, but a giant leap in saving women's lives.

Had I recognised the symptoms, I might be writing a different book today - one of survival.

Chapter 1

Early beginnings

I admit it freely - I was ignorant. I did not have a clue. I have racked my brains and I still cannot even recall knowing anyone who has had ovarian cancer. I had no point of reference to judge by. I had no idea what the symptoms were. And worst of all, even if I did recognise some of the more obvious ones, I doubt I would have taken them that seriously. I had a totally blasé attitude to cancer, which I suppose is hardly surprising when you consider that this was the third time I had contracted the disease. Previously, I was diagnosed with bladder cancer followed some years later by breast cancer.

It all started in 1995 when I was fifty-two years of age and as fit as a butcher's dog. I had, until then, never had a day's serious illness in my life, and hardly knew my doctor. Hospitals to me were alien places that you only went to when visiting family or friends. They were not places where you ever envisaged spending time as a patient. But that was all to change.

The first indication I had that something might be wrong was in September 1995. I seemed to be passing more urine that usual. Thinking that I had a slight infection - this was the only symptom - I didn't bother going to the doctor and convinced myself that it would clear up naturally without the need for drugs. A month later it was still there and I came to the conclusion that it was cystitis. I knew what the symptoms were - my sister-in-law suffered from it. The main one was frequently passing urine. I also knew that it could be easily cleared up with a course of antibiotics. With this in mind, I made an appointment for the next day to see one of the doctors at the practice where I was registered. My visit to the doctor was painless. She took a urine test, said I had a mild infection which was probably cystitis, and gave me a prescription for a ten-day course of antibiotics. Four days later the infection was cleared up, but I continued to take the tablets to make sure that it did not return

Two weeks later, after I had finished the tablets, it was back again. The doctor had told me that if it returned, I should go back and see her, so another appointment was made. This time she gave me a stronger dose of antibiotics and urged me to return immediately if these new tablets did not clear it up.

It soon became clear that it was not cystitis. It had come back again, so I made my third appointment to see the doctor, wondering what it could be, but not concerned that it might be serious. The doctor decided that further investigation was needed and arranged for me to see an urologist at Putney Hospital. An appointment was made for early November, six weeks away. I would have preferred an earlier one as it was proving to be a bit of a nuisance running to the loo all the time.

On the day of the appointment I saw a young doctor who said that I needed to come back for tests and to see the consultant urologist. Another appointment was made for late November when I would have an endoscopy. I was still not worried and believed that I had no cause for concern.

I cannot remember much about that Thursday afternoon. It must have been just an ordinary day, like any other. There was nothing momentous about it that would make it stick in my mind. I struggle even now to think back to it, but nothing comes to mind.

The hospital, on Putney Common, is not far from where I live in Barnes. I used public transport instead of driving because I did not want the problem of finding somewhere to park. The clinic was nearly empty when I arrived and the test was done fairly fast. I was ignorant of hospital systems and unaware of the long waits that are part of the NHS, so the speed of the test and consultation meant nothing to me. I accepted it as normal.

The consultant urologist, whose name I cannot remember, came to see me in the cubicle, where he had asked me to wait. A middle-aged man, all that I remember about him was that he had kind brown eyes. I was sitting in the chair by the bed and he sat himself down on the bed. Looking at me, he said: "You have a tumour on your bladder that needs to be removed." For some reason that I cannot explain, I asked him if it were cancerous, although I did not have any thoughts of cancer in my head. I was astonished when he said yes.

"It is not serious and is very treatable," he said, seeing the look of surprise on my face. "People live for years with this. You will probably die of something else," he added reassuringly.

He then went on to say that I could have the operation in January, but if I were concerned about waiting, he would re-arrange his diary and do it within the next two weeks.

It was getting close to Christmas and I decided that if it were not that serious, I would wait until the New Year. He assured me that another two or three weeks would not make that much difference.

An operation at this time would have upset my Christmas arrangements. My husband (his name is Vincent - but I call him Vincey), and I were spending Christmas with our daughter, Jacqueline who lives in Madrid with her husband and baby daughter. I had already booked the tickets and I was reluctant to make any change to our existing plans. We were both looking forward to spending our first Christmas with our granddaughter, who was only a month old. It would have taken wild horses to keep me away from Madrid.

Thanking the consultant, I said January would be fine. He explained that I would get a letter confirming the date of admission to the hospital and I was not to worry. "I have lots of patients with the same complaint and they live into their eighties and nineties," he said. I left the hospital feeling that while I might have cancer, it did not seem too bad.

I was not looking forward to telling my husband. He hates it when there is anything wrong with Jackie or me. When I got home and told him, he was very upset. And although I tried to reassure him, telling him that it sounded much worse than it was, he was not having it. I explained that the doctor envisaged no problems when he removed the tumour, but he did not believe me. Within minutes he was on the phone to our daughter telling her everything. And within hours, the news had spread across three countries, Britain, Spain and Ireland. Everyone is remembering the death of my sister eight years previously from cancer.

Soon the whole family knows and the phone is ringing continuously, everyone demanding to know what is happening.

There are four of us - three girls and a boy. Me, I am the eldest, followed by Pauline, next our brother Pierce and finally Frances, the baby of the family. But it felt like fifty thousand as each one interrogated me individually. I had to repeat every word the doctor said, why I agreed to wait until after Christmas instead of having it done immediately and could we trust the doctor - what were the guarantees.

Jackie soon joins Vincey, Pauline and Frances in demanding that I get another opinion. They are finding my attitude too laid back. To their way of thinking I have cancer and there is no such thing as a good cancer. The only one that took the news calmly was my brother Pierce. He believed me when I said that it was not that serious. What none of them could forget was that our sister Pearl had died of breast cancer at the young age of thirty-four.

I was feeling very guilty that I was upsetting everyone's Christmas and kept telling them that there was nothing to worry about. But instead of listening to me, they stopped talking about it in front of me and discussed it amongst themselves instead. I was to learn later that they thought I was trying to convince myself that everything was normal, when in fact it was far from normal. I had cancer.

Why they should have thought that I was refusing to accept that I had cancer, I don't know. I am a very ordinary, practical sort of person and I like things to be straightforward. I don't like bad news to be dressed in frills or coated in honey - I like it straight.

But despite my protestations and attempts to convince them that things were not as bad as they seemed, the news put a damper on everyone's Christmas. We had been so looking forward to Christmas with our new granddaughter, our daughter and our son-in-law, Gilberto. But everyone was behaving as though they were walking on eggshells and while I understood, it did not make it any easier. After a while I gave up trying to explain that this was different and the doctor was very confident that I would be OK. There was no need for all this misery, I kept telling them. This was treatable. And unlike breast cancer, there was even a possibility that it would go away.

But all my attempts were in vain. There was no consoling them. I think they were all waiting for the news that the operation would not be successful and the only thing after that was death. I know this makes them all sound like drama queens, yet nothing could be further from the truth. It was only when I started to lose patience with them and told them to forget it - they were not getting rid of me that easily - that they started to calm down. Somehow, it eased the intensity of the situation and everyone decided to stand back and wait for the outcome.

Yet despite all the misery, we enjoyed five wonderful days in Madrid. We took our granddaughter out daily - even Christmas Day - to the lovely, big, park close to where my daughter lives.

Madrid can be cold in winter, but unlike London, it is not damp, so trips to the park were quite pleasant. The red squirrels, which are in abundance and almost tame, followed us each day in the hope of getting some titbits. Once we got used to them, we came prepared with bread. My daughter could not understand why there was never any bread in the house, yet hardly anyone ate it. She did not realise that she was feeding the local wildlife.

On one of our visits to the park, Vincey had the grand idea of taking our granddaughter, Natalia, on a trip around the Prada, one of Spain's most famous museums, and just a five-minute walk from the park. But we decided against the idea almost as quickly as he'd thought of it. What if she started bawling her head off as we walked her around the beautifully decorated rooms filled with the work of some of the most famous painters in the world? We decided that at this age, food and sleep were her greatest priorities. Appreciation of art could come later.

The days sped by and soon we were at the airport. Our flight home on New Year's Eve was delayed. I cannot remember why or for how long, but I remember wishfully thinking that perhaps we were meant to stay in Spain. I hated leaving my daughter and granddaughter behind. So did Vincey.

Chapter 2

Looming close

Back in London and with Christmas and the New Year a distant memory, I found my mind wandering in the direction of the hospital and thinking what my stay there would be like. It was not that I was concerned, more curious. I didn't know how long I would have to stay in; I was expecting two, maybe three days. The last time I had been in hospital was when my daughter was born, nearly four decades ago, so I had no idea what to expect. All I knew was that it was looming closer.

On the day, I arrived at Putney Hospital on a Sunday afternoon and with the least amount of fuss was shown to a bed in a ward that had one other empty bed. An hour later a pleasant young woman doctor came to see me. She went through all the usual questions, took my blood pressure and told me how brave I was. I didn't feel very brave and my first reaction was suspicion. Had I not been given all of the information correctly and was the situation much worse than I had been led to believe, I was asking myself. When I asked her what had changed since I had last seen the consultant, she replied that nothing had changed.

So why do I need to be brave? I asked her. Now aware that I had misunderstood her remarks as something more sinister, she said that I must be brave because I was so calm, not creating a fuss. Perhaps I should have been more concerned, I told myself, but then put the thought out of my head. There was no point worrying about it now. She then went on to explain what would happen the next day: the anaesthetist would be along to see me in the morning, as would the consultant who would do the operation. It was at this point that I discovered the fate of my poor consultant with the kind brown eyes.

Apparently, he had been on his way home to Southampton just before Christmas when his car skidded on black ice. He was now in hospital in a coma and on a life support machine and was unlikely ever to practice medicine again. I found out later that he had partly recovered and because of his vast knowledge and experience, had become a lecturer. I remember thinking at the time what a loss to humanity. Life, as we know, is not fair.

With all of the paperwork completed, the doctor left saying she would see me in the morning. I rang Vincey, as promised, and assured him that everything was OK and that I would be having my operation the following afternoon. He said he would be up to see me in the morning, but I asked him to wait until the afternoon when the operation was over. He agreed.

The bush telegraph was working overtime and within ten minutes of speaking to my husband, my daughter and my two sisters were on the telephone. They had all rung to check that everything was OK. Frances, who had come over from Dublin, was staying with Pauline in Hampshire, where she lives. When I spoke to Pauline I knew she had been crying, I could still hear it in her voice.

Monday morning dawned bright, but cold. With *nil by mouth* - an expression that never fails to amuse me for no reason that I can think of - decorating the head of my bed, the food trolley gave me a wide berth. No breakfast for me - not even a drink of water. Once the usual procedures of blood pressure and temperature were over, I considered going for a walk outside to get some fresh air - the ward was hot to the point of suffocation. But I changed my mind when, looking through the French doors, I saw the grass was covered in frost. Instead I went to the morning room, which was slightly cooler. About an hour later - I was starting to lose track of time - a nurse came and told me that the anaesthetist was on his way and I should return to the ward. His main concern was how

I would react to the anaesthetic. I had never had opiates pumped into my body before so I was not sure what my reaction would be either. But I suddenly remembered someone I knew had told me that anaesthetics had made her sick. I sincerely hoped that was not going to be the case with me.

I was scheduled to go down to the operating theatre at, as far as I can remember, about one thirty. I would have murdered for a cup of tea. I'd had nothing to eat **or** drink since midnight and I was wishing that it were all over so that I could have some food. I was starving

It's not strictly true to call it an operation. You are not cut. But it is performed in an operating theatre under general anaesthetic. I suppose the nearest to it is keyhole surgery, in that there is no wound. It is described as non-invasive surgery. To remove the cancer tumours from my bladder, an instrument is slipped inside that scrapes the tumours from the bladder wall.

I was oblivious to all this. I remember them taking me down on the gurney to the room next to the operating theatre where they administer the drugs. A needle was inserted into a vein in the back of my hand. Into this were fed the drugs. As I had never had an anaesthetic before, I was not prepared for the wonderful, relaxing sensation that spread through my body. That was the last thing I remember.

My next recollection was when I woke up back in the ward and Vincey is sitting beside me. Apart from feeling a bit groggy from the residue of the anaesthetic, I felt fine. After I have moved about a bit to see if everything was in working order and to see if I felt any pain, I was curious to know why I have a tube with a bag on the end of it attached to me.

The nurse, seeing that I am awake, came over and asked me if I was all right and if I would like something to eat and drink. My reply: *Is the pope a Catholic* caused some confusion. She was Asian. But had no trouble understanding and within ten minutes was back with a mug of hot tea and some toast.

An hour later the consultant comes to see me. These doctors really work long hours. He has been in the hospital since eight o'clock this morning and is still here at seven o'clock in the evening. He said that everything had gone well - the tumours had been removed and all that I now needed was for my bladder to be washed with a radiation-based substance that would cauterise the bladder wound and reduce the frequency of the tumours returning. This would take about an hour and would be administered using the catheter - my mysterious tube with the bag attached. He said it would be done in the morning and I could go home immediately afterwards. I was to have many of these in the years ahead and I christened the substance my nuclear fuel.

An appointment would be made for me to return in six months' time for a check up, he said. Other than that I was fine. I thanked him for everything and said I would see him at the appointed time.

I had spent less that 48 hours in hospital. Cancer had been removed from my body. The worst part of the entire exercise was the boredom of sitting around waiting for things to happen. Is it any wonder that I treated the disease so casually? It would have been more painful to have an ingrown toenail removed, I suspected.

The following six months were perfectly normal. No aches, no pains, nothing. It was as if I had dreamt the whole thing. I did not feel any different.

My next appointment, which had been made for the day care unit in Queen Mary's, Roehampton, proved to be fast and trouble-free, but I was not happy when they told me that the tumours were back again. They were smaller than the previous ones, but still had to be removed.

Three weeks later I was back in the day care unit for my operation. My appointment was for two o'clock. I had been told to neither eat nor drink from six o'clock in the morning: otherwise they would not be able to do the operation. By two thirty I was on my way to the operating theatre and by four thirty I was back in the ward, awake and enjoying tea and toast. At five thirty I left in a taxi accompanied by Vincey. When I got home, I prepared dinner for both of us. The only difference was that I went to bed earlier than usual. Next day I was back in the office as if nothing had happened. I have to say I only have praise for the efficiency of these units. I have attended them for many years now and they are probably the most efficient part of the National Health Service. It goes to show what can be done. Unfortunately, it also makes you wonder why there are such bottlenecks elsewhere.

This routine became part of my life for the next two years. The tumours were returning regularly and I was having operations every six months. I have to admit that I gave no serious thought to the whole procedure. I had two appointments and two operations a year.

About this time, Jackie started to question the frequency with which the tumours were returning. It was obvious that I had a high recurrence level and she wanted to know if there was any other reason for this. She asked me to get my file from my GP and from the hospital so that she could pass them to an urologist friend of my son-in-law's family in the US.

A couple of weeks later, he gave my daughter his verdict. Yes, I did have a high recurrence rate, but I was receiving the standard treatment for that particular cancer. However, he suggested that I should ask for BCG tablets, which would reduce the frequency of the tumours.

At my very next appointment - yes it was back again - I asked the consultant if I could have these tablets. He said that it would be better for me to have what I called my nuclear fuel - I had not had it after the past three operations - as the tablets could make me sick. He said he would make sure that it was done after my next operation.

The regular use of the nuclear fuel certainly did the trick. Now that my bladder was washed after every operation, the tumours suddenly started re-appearing only once a year, much to my delight. Even more surprising and very welcome, a few years later, they disappeared altogether. I have not had any treatment for the past four years. Although I will have to continue having annual check ups for the next six years, if after ten years I am still clear, they will accept that the cancer may not come back.

All those years ago, my consultant with the kind brown eyes had told me that in some cases - few in number - the cancer could actually disappear, never to return. I thought he was trying to cheer me up at the time, but I am hoping that he will be proved right.

Is it any wonder that I am blasé about cancer? Over all those years, I only had one scare and that was when a doctor doing the operation thought that she had punctured my bladder wall. She hadn't.

Chapter 3

Knocked over with a feather

When I was diagnosed with breast cancer in 2001, you could have knocked me over with a feather. No one was more surprised than me. To begin with, it was little short of a miracle that I found out when I did. For years my doctor had been sending me letters urging me to make an appointment for a mammogram. But I ignored them. Why, I don't know. You would have thought that with my sister dying of breast cancer that would have been incentive enough.

All I know is that if I had not made the appointment - helped in no small way by Vincey asking me daily if I had done it - I would not have known about the cancer as quickly or as early as I did. I would not have been in a position to be able to take preventative measures. It's not that I like to put my head in the sand and pretend that everything is OK. If there is a problem, I like to know about it and take measures to solve it, but I never ever thought that there was a possibility that I would get breast cancer, which is pretty stupid when you think that it is already in the family.

I had an appointment for about three thirty on a Wednesday afternoon in August at one of those big mobile trailer-type lorries that travel around the country. It was parked in the grounds of Roehampton Hospital, where I was to present myself.

My two grandchildren - Jackie had another daughter nearly six years previously - were staying with us at the time so I arranged for my friend Rosemary to take them to the cinema while I was having the test done.

I drove down to the hospital - it only takes about ten minutes, and went to the mobile unit. There was a short wait, then the test, which took about ten minutes. I was back home within forty minutes and I never gave it another thought.

Imagine my surprise when a couple of weeks later Vincey rings me at the office one morning to tell me a letter has arrived from the Breast Clinic that is attached to St. George's Hospital in Tooting. They want to take another look and asked me to confirm that I accepted the appointment.

Some weeks later Vincey and I turned up at the clinic. They did another mammogram and said they were sure that everything was OK, but there was just something there that they would like to investigate further. They showed us the film from the mammogram and kept pointing to small white irregular-shaped dots that looked like tiny clouds to me. There were lots of them and they all looked the same, but the doctor kept pointing to a couple that she thought was suspect.

"We need to do a biopsy," she said, and arranged for me to come back the following Thursday. They said that as there was a history of breast cancer in the family and it can be hereditary, best to double check. Understandably, I was becoming concerned. So was Vincey.

For the rest of the week I kept trying to put it out of my mind. There was no point worrying until I knew whether I had something to worry about or not. The following Thursday, we arrived at the clinic for the third time. For no reason that I could identify, we had to wait ages. Eventually, they called me thorough to the room where they do the tests. There were a couple of nurses and a woman doctor, all very sympathetic. They tried to be as reassuring as possible, telling me that this was just a precaution and it did not mean that I had cancer. Lots of women had it done, they said, and it usually proved that there was nothing to be concerned about.

When they do the test, they put you in the position as if they were doing a mammogram - it is like been in a vice - and stick a very large needle into your breast to remove the tissue. You have to stand very still, so that they can accurately target the part where they suspect the cancer cells are. This is very painful and they had to do it a number of times before they were satisfied with the results.

All this took about three-quarters of an hour. Afterwards, they made another appointment for the following Thursday, when I should return for the results. We went home, both of us feeling pretty miserable and wondering what the outcome would be.

We also had another task that neither of us was looking forward to - informing the family. Up to now we had said nothing to them and we would have preferred to keep it that way, but it was looking more and more as if the result was positive, so we decided to get it over with. Remembering the great upset years before when I was diagnosed with bladder cancer, we knew that this was going to prove to be much more difficult. Calm was only restored at the time when everyone realised that the bladder cancer was treatable and not life threatening. And now here we were again - telling everyone that I had suspected breast cancer. There was no glossing over this and trying to minimise the impact. Everyone in the family was aware of the potential of this cancer to kill, which made it much worse. I have come to the conclusion that cancer is probably the one disease that causes such distress in families. It was certainly causing it in mine.

Of all the family, I hated telling my daughter the most. And, not surprisingly, it proved to be the most difficult. She tries to be so brave and supportive. As I write this, I am remembering that day and the tears are streaming down my face. I cannot continue, so I go to the kitchen and make myself a cup of tea. Fifteen minutes later I am back in front of the computer trying to pick up where I left off.

As the cancer has not been confirmed yet, I am still hoping that it is a mistake and that the little white clouds are not cancer cells, but calcium. I am also starting to wonder how I have managed to get cancer twice. Do I have the cancer gene? I don't even know what it is, only what I have been reading in the newspapers. Scientists have discovered that there is a cancer gene. Surely if you get cancer twice you must have it, I reasoned.

The wait to the following Thursday for the results proved to be long and worrying, but I would know for definite. There were no further tests I could have - I either had it or I hadn't. As we set out for the clinic, I tried to be as calm as possible so as not to upset Vincey. But I was feeling very apprehensive and would have preferred to be going anywhere, but the clinic.

Once there, we were seen fairly quickly. The doctor put the film in the lightbox on the wall and pointed to those little white clouds again - yes, they were cancerous, she said. The biopsy had come back positive. They needed to be removed. I felt sick when I saw the worried look on Vincey's face. He seemed to suffer more than I did. But in the middle of all this gloom, there was good news. It was not full blown cancer, but a low-grade variant that was non-invasive. If I were going to get breast cancer, this was the best one to have. And it had been identified at such an early stage that it could be treated fast and effectively and without the usual horrors of breast removal, chemotherapy, radiotherapy or any other long periods of medication.

To my way of thinking, this was an action replay of the conversation I had at Putney Hospital all those years ago with the consultant with the kind brown eyes when he told me that the bladder cancer I had was treatable and I would probably die of something else. I cheered up immediately and while we waited for them to do the paperwork for me to attend the breast clinic at Queen Mary's, Roehampton, I voiced my thoughts to Vincey. I could see that he desperately wanted to believe me, but he felt that I was being too optimistic. The nurse who brought me the card with my appointment for the hospital said: "I would never have thought that you had cancer." I have to admit, I felt a lot more cheerful on the journey home. I spoke to my daughter, my sisters and my brother explaining that it was not as bad as first thought and there was no need for worry. Typically, no one believed me.

Rosemary rang later and I explained everything. She had suffered breast cancer herself about ten years previously and was very aware of the effects of full-blown breast cancer. She first got it when her twins were only two years old. It proved to be very traumatic for her with such young children, but they removed the lump and she was fine. Then, one day, short of the magic five years - the thinking at that time was that if you survived five years it was unlikely to return - it was back. This time they removed the breast. Having experienced cancer twice, she understood how I was feeling and was very supportive.

I was becoming fed-up with hospitals, clinics, doctors and nurses - the whole paraphernalia of cancer and its treatment. I was fed-up with being pulled around, thrust into machines, keeping appointments - I wished I had never heard of the disease. I know this all sounds ungrateful when these people were trying to help, but that was how I felt.

My next appointment was for a couple of weeks' time. I don't even remember the day. I just know the month was October. I had put the whole thing out of my mind. I would think about it again nearer the time. I had no reason to believe that I would be told anything different at the clinic.

As usual, Vincey accompanied me and we arrived at the clinic far too early. I think it is much worse for the men than the women. I see them sitting there - not sure what to do - waiting to hear what is going to happen next and looking totally bewildered by it all. While you are dealing with the problem and giving it your attention, they are doing their best to be supportive, but judging by the expressions on their faces they seem to feel totally divorced from what is happening. So they just sit there not sure what to do. I try to discourage Vincey from attending appointments with me, but

I am seldom successful. He is convinced that I always play down the seriousness of what is happening and only tell him part of the truth because I don't want to upset him. There is an element of truth in what he says.

Queen Mary's breast cancer clinic is a mad house. Sometimes, there are far too many patients and you can wait anything up to two hours to see a consultant. Other times, you can wait about ten minutes. There is neither rhyme nor reason for the delays and asking the staff is a waste of time. They have standard replies, which they dish out to everyone. It is hard to gauge whether the problem is a lack of doctors to the number of patients, poor management of resources or what. What I do know is that people suffering from cancer could do without the stress of these clinics and the length of time they have to wait.

I have an appointment to see a Mr Cummins. I did not have to wait long, it just seemed an age because we had arrived far too early. He turned out to be a very pleasant and rather laid back Australian. He confirmed everything that I had been told at the clinic in Tooting and said that I would have the operation at Kingston Hospital within a month. He emphasised that it was not a matter for concern because it had been diagnosed so early and once the cells had been removed, there should no longer be a problem. This was all good news and exactly what I wanted to hear. I explained that I was due for my bladder check up soon. He said that I should see my consultant as soon as possible and if there were any tumours to be removed, he would arrange it with my consultant at Kingston, whom he knew, so that both operations could be done together.

Within a week, I had both of my appointments - one in the day care unit for my bladder and another for the operation. The day care appointment was for a Friday. I was in and out within forty minutes with the all clear. It was a relief that I needed no treatment. My next stop in a couple of weeks' time was back here - in the main part of the hospital for my operation. This was to be a first for me - I had never had a proper operation in my life before.

Chapter 4

Operation Kingston, Surrey that is

I have little recollection of my arrival at Kingston Hospital for my breast cancer operation. By now I am becoming a hospital junkie and I no longer retain information on arrivals and departures. My visits are becoming too frequent to remember. I know it was a Monday and that it was in November and that I had to ring the hospital at four pm to confirm that there had been no emergencies and a bed was still available. I probably remember ringing the hospital because I had never been asked to do this before. Bag packed - my weekend bag was seeing hospitals with much the same regularity as me and, like me was becoming a bit frayed at the edges. I set off on my trek to Kingston Hill, where the hospital is located.

Kingston is a general hospital. I think that it used to be a cottage hospital at some stage. But those days are now long gone. It acquired a large number of patients when Queen Mary's in Roehampton closed its wards and its doors to the sick and needy. Kingston is being extended at a dramatic rate. There are bricklayers, electricians, plumbers, cement lorries, cranes reaching up to the sky - all the paraphernalia of a building site - everywhere. I remember thinking that if they continued to expand at this pace, they would soon be one of the biggest hospitals ever and be spread over the entire county of Surrey.

On arrival, I went through the usual procedures and, once installed, rang Vincey to tell him that everything was OK. The operation, I was told, was planned for the next day, but no time was specified, so I was in the dark as to when it would be performed.

I knew that I had to have the area identified for the surgical team. The quickest and easiest way to do this was for the doctor down in the X-ray department to do a very tight and close mammogram, highlight where the cancer cells were and then draw a line around the area so that the surgeon would know where to cut.

Apparently the cells were in an awkward place and I remember that she took a long time to get it exactly right so that everything would be removed. She was a lovely lady and I saw her again when I went back for my check up. Her insistence on correctly identifying the area to the nth degree resulted in my getting the all clear.

I was now ready for the operation and back with my friend - *nil by mouth* - decorating the head of my bed. The anaesthetist came to see me, a young man of Middle Eastern or Asian background. He was very reassuring and went through the procedure with me, asking if I was allergic to anything. He said he would insert a particular type of drip so that I could use it later to activate a painkiller should I be in any pain after the operation. Then off he went, saying he would see me tomorrow.

The following morning dawned reasonably bright for November - not the sort of day that you would want to be in hospital. With nothing to do I wandered around looking for the trolley with the newspapers, but I was too early. Then it was time to go down to X-ray to have my breast marked. I was back again on the ward within the hour. The nurse came over to my bed to see if everything had gone OK and said that she needed to go through the checklist with me before I went down to the operating theatre. Together we ticked all the relevant boxes and agreed that everything was as it should be.

It must have been about twelve o'clock when I eventually went down to theatre, but I'm not sure. It is so easy to lose track of time in hospitals. The anaesthetist was there waiting and a nurse put a line into a vein in the back of my hand. Then there was that wonderful flush running through my body and I don't remember anything until I woke up about five hours later. Vincey was sitting beside my bed. His life with me seems to be spent either attending or visiting me in hospitals. He finds it very stressful, but he never complains. I try to convince him that it is not necessary for him to visit or accompany me to every hospital or clinic. Sometimes he agrees, but mostly he is there with me.

I was very, very drowsy and could not keep awake. I kept dosing off. This was not normal for me. I usually recover quite quickly. But not this time. I don't know how long my husband had been sitting there, but I kept telling him to go home. Now that he could see that I was OK, he agreed. Just as he was leaving, Rosemary arrived. I remember trying to talk to her, but there seemed to be big gaps in the conversation and I said that there was little point in her staying as I was continuing to fall asleep in the middle of a conversation. She told me this later. I have no recollection of any of it.

A couple of hours later, I was beginning to wake up and was looking for the instrument that was supposed to allow me to control any pain I might have. But I could not find it. It was not that I was in pain, I just wanted to see what it looked like - I had never had anything like this fitted before. Calling the nurse, I asked her where it was. She said it had not been fitted because I was sensitive to opiates. This immediately set the alarm bells ringing. I knew I was not sensitive to opiates - I'd had them too many times not to know their effect on me. My immediate reaction was one of disbelief. Then I realised that she was lying. What was most worrying was the glibness of the lie. She did it with such ease - it was almost like second nature to her. If I had not known better, I would have believed her. And she was the nurse that was looking after me. Everything she said to me from then on was taken with a big pinch of salt. The anaesthetist had been a little heavy-handed, which explained why I had been having difficulty waking up properly and why I did not want anything to eat or drink.

I dosed off again and did not wake up properly until early next morning. I was hungry and parched. It is useful having a facility in a ward to make tea and toast, one that I immediately took advantage of. For the next few hours I lay in bed reading. I felt fine - just a little soreness where I had been cut - and was keen to go home. But I was not sure what the reaction was going to be when I asked. The surgeon who had done the operation and his entourage arrived to do their rounds about eleven o'clock. He asked how I was and seemed surprised that I wanted to go home, but said that he saw no reason why I should not. By late afternoon I was back home.

Thursday was a pleasant day. With little or nothing to do, Vincey and I just lazed around, read the papers and finally decided that instead of cooking, we would go out to lunch. It was very enjoyable, but I got a bit carried away with the wine and came home feeling a little light-headed. Friday morning I was back in the office. The wound was a little sore, but other than that there was no indication that I had had breast cancer.

Two weeks later I went to the breast cancer clinic at Queen Mary's, Roehampton, to have my stitches removed and see if I needed further treatment or medication. I saw the consultant John Cummins. When I had first seen him nearly two months previously, he had told me that he would oversee the operation. Now he went through everything - were the stitches hurting? How did I feel? Was I back at work? Was there anything I was concerned about? I told him I felt fine and asked if there was anything I should be doing. He said no, but I could have a course of radiotherapy if I wanted it. I asked him if I needed it and he said no, so I declined. There was no mention of the link between breast cancer and ovarian cancer, but I was told to come back in six months for a mammogram.

I had been diagnosed with low grade, non-invasive breast cancer. It had been detected early enough to be successfully treated. And because it was *in situ*, it would not jump to other parts of the body, which is what can happen with other breast cancers. As far as they could tell, all the cancer cells had been removed. I felt fine and I needed no further treatment. I would have to come back once a year for a check-up, but other than that it was almost as if I had never had the disease. Was it any wonder that I had a blasé attitude to cancer? Was it any wonder that my blasé attitude was growing in confidence.

Chapter 5

First hint of something wrong

In August 2002 I was feeling good and decided that as I was nearing sixty it was time to make changes to my life. I would complete all the things that I had started. But it took me until February 2003 before I took any positive action. I had been working for a dot com for a number of years, but now I wanted a new challenge. A couple of years earlier I had started to write a book. A work of fiction, it was about a new political party fighting a general election on a manifesto that was totally different from anything the existing parties had to offer. I think I had completed about one hundred thousand words and I wanted the time to finish it. I also wanted to create a Website for women of fifty plus. Women in this age group are invisible in today's youth dominated society. I wanted to make them visible. I wanted to get them involved in all sorts of activities that would heighten their profile and give them equal billing with men of the same age. This is a hobby of mine, probably based on my attitude to age and life, neither one should be seen as a barrier to doing things.

In my mind, I don't feel old - whatever that is supposed to mean. I can't run as fast as I used to and my days of racing up and down the stairs are numbered: now I am forced to walk. But I am fit and active. I go to the gym three times a week - every Monday, Wednesday and Friday morning.

I am interested in most of what is happening around me, but my biggest fascination is for information technology, particularly computers. I accept that the young are far better at using computers than I am - I only have to see my two granddaughters to know that.

They whiz around computers as if they were born programmed to use them.

Most of my life I have been an achiever. When I set my sights on something, I go after it. I am not saying that I am always successful, but I will give it my best shot. When I decided early in life that I wanted to be a journalist, that is what I did. And as part of that job, I travelled the world extensively, reporting from trade zones to war zones and enjoyed every minute of it. But now I had a new challenge and there was no doubt in my mind that I would succeed. I wanted to finish my book and create my own Website, so I set myself a schedule. My new part-time hours meant that I could spend two days writing and one day creating the design and preparing the content for the site.

I don't know when I first started to notice it - it must have been about a month into my new work schedule. Everything seemed to be taking much longer than it should. The reason was obvious - once I thought about it - I was not working properly. I noticed that I would come back from the gym, have breakfast and instead of starting work, I would sit in the kitchen reading the paper. I found every excuse not to work.

At about this time I also noticed that I was not feeling one hundred per cent. Despite my various ailments, I always felt fit and well. It was nothing that I could put my finger on, just a general feeling of not being well - a lack of energy, a lack of motivation.

I ignored it and decided that it must be my age catching up with me. Then I started to get heartburn. The last time I'd had heartburn was when I was pregnant over forty years ago. I ignored that too. Part of the ageing process, I thought. It was only when I started to get tummy ache that I decided to go to the doctor, but I waited a couple of months before I actually got around to making the appointment. I never get tummy ache. If by chance I do, I can usually identify the reason - constipation or something equally innocuous. I monitored the ache - tried to see if there was a pattern to it. Did it happen when I ate a particular food? Was it at any particular time - in the mornings, in the evenings, when I went to bed, when I got up? Was it when I exercised - walking long distances or overdoing it at the gym? There was no pattern. After much thought I decided that because it was so mild, it could not be that serious. But it was persistent and I was still continuing to feel under the weather, so I rang the doctor and made an appointment.

I went to see her sometime in early September. She did the usual tests - blood pressure and blood - both OK. She asked me if I wanted to be fast-tracked and I said no, I did not feel that ill. An appointment eventually arrived to attend a clinic at Queen Mary's, Roehampton in November. I continued to go to the office on my appointed days and to the gym. Everything was much the same as usual. I made no changes to my lifestyle. I ate the same foods, continued with the same activities and tried to concentrate on my book and my Website. I have to admit I was not making much progress on either.

In November I attended the clinic and was seen by a charming young doctor in his early thirties who said he could find no reason why I should be having either heartburn or tummy ache. He sent me off for a scan and twenty minutes later I was back with him for the result. It showed nothing. He then suggested that I have this test - I won't go into detail - but it was horrible. Basically, they wanted to see if I had bowel cancer. I had the test a couple of weeks later and no cancer was found, but I did have that most common of diseases affecting a large part of the population over fifty - diverticulosis.

It is rampant in western or industrialised countries where the diet contains too little roughage. It is usually to be found in the lower abdomen and most people are unaware that they have it. But it can become a problem if the area becomes inflamed. I now had a reason for my tummy ache, or so I believed. The heartburn, I decided, must be an ageing thing. It was suggested that I heal the diverticulosis by diet rather than medication and an appointment was made for me to see a dietician. This proved to be a waste of time.

The foods she suggested that I ate were already part of our daily diet. We had changed our eating habits years before when Vincey had triple bypasses. We ate very little processed food - preparing all our own meals, ate hardly any animal fat and were generally aware of what to avoid. The main part of our diet was fresh fruit and vegetables, although we slipped from time to time and ate chips, chocolate, cake and all those other lovely, but forbidden foods. But generally, there was nothing in my diet that I could change that would make a difference.

There seemed to be nowhere else to go either. According to the tests, there was nothing wrong. For the rest of 2003 I still felt as if I had no energy, but I was getting used to it. We went to Madrid for Christmas and I was able to go to the park with the children - I now had a delightful grandson - play football and chase them around, but I found I was out of breath much quicker than usual. I was still going to the gym and did not notice anything different.

When we were in Madrid, Jackie asked me if Alexandra, the second eldest of our grandchildren could come and stay with us. The children are bi-lingual, speaking both Spanish and English like natives, but my daughter thought that Alexandra would benefit from more exposure to the English language, so it was decided that she would come to us in April, once her exams were over. She arrived in mid-April travelling as an accompanied minor - one of the hostesses took care of her - escorting her on to the aircraft and looking after her until she was collected. We went out to Heathrow Airport to pick her up and, as usual, we were miles too early - Vincey believes in getting to airports and hospitals with plenty of time to spare in case there are any unforeseen problems. I make no allowance for such delays and have sometimes come very close to chasing aircraft down the runway to catch a flight.

Alexandra is eleven years old and you would hardly know she was there. She is wonderful and settled in immediately. The children are used to London - they come here a lot. But on this occasion it proved to be rather unfortunate for the child that she happened to arrive in London just as I was stumbling into what was to prove to be the worst illness I have ever had in my life

The next time I noticed that something was not quite right was at the end of April, five months after my tests. Rosemary and I always take each other out to dinner on the nearest Saturday to our birthdays. It has become something of a tradition. It was my birthday and on this particular occasion my sister Pauline, who lives in Hampshire, decided to join us. A new Chinese restaurant had opened close by and we decided to try it.

We made a wise choice - the food was delicious - light - more like Thai food, but with that particular Chinese flavour. At the end of the evening, I was feeling very uncomfortable and could hardly sit up straight. It was not that I had eaten or drunk too much. But I felt as if I had something pulling at one of my lungs and it was being dragged down. I had to keep straightening my back to relieve the ache. The next day it was gone and I forgot about it.

A week later, on Thursday, the sixth of May, I noticed that my stomach was even more swollen than usual and I was feeling very uncomfortable. My back was aching and I did not want to eat. I decided that a visit to the doctor was needed and made an appointment for the next day.

I have a lovely lady doctor who was most sympathetic After she did her usual checks - she listened to my tummy, said that it was wind and gave me a prescription for tablets that would ease it. I picked up the tablets straight away and started to take them on the Friday afternoon. I went to the gym on Monday, as usual. I noticed no change in my tummy - it was not going down, but I continued to take the tablets.

During this time I was getting emails from Jackie in Madrid telling me about a woman in the United States who had died of ovarian cancer. It was not that she knew much about ovarian cancer - she was getting the emails from a friend in the US who was telling her what the symptoms were - similar to mine - in particular the swollen tummy. The friend was also telling her about a blood test - the CA125 - now one of the recognised tests that confirm whether women are suffering from ovarian cancer or not. Jackie kept telling me to ask the doctor for the test to be done, but I was reluctant for no reason that I can justify. I suppose I did not believe that I had cancer and I did not want to upset the doctor by not seeming to believe her, so I kept putting it off. Despite two bouts of cancer - another indication of my attitude - I had not even considered it could be that.

Tuesday morning, as I was getting dressed to go to the office, I noticed a definite change that I could no longer ignore - my tummy was getting even bigger. I had worn the same pair of trousers the previous week, but I could not get the zip to go up. This was worrying and I decided to go and see the doctor immediately the surgery was open.

I saw the doctor who owns the practice - he is my husband's doctor - and he took blood and said he would send it off to the laboratory. He gave me a prescription for a urine infection, but admitted that it was unlikely that this was what was causing the problem. He suggested that I ring on Thursday morning for the results and keep my appointment to see my own doctor on Friday.

On Wednesday morning, I went to the gym for what proved to be the last time. It was an attempt to keep my life normal. Back home, I ate my breakfast - the last meal I was to have for nearly two weeks. My tummy was getting bigger and bigger and I was becoming more and more uncomfortable. I did not feel hungry for the rest of the day. I would just sip some lemonade or water, but I could eat nothing solid. I even had difficulty drinking my favourite tipple - tea. During this time Jackie was repeatedly asking me to have a CA125. She said I needed it done, even if it were only to eliminate the possibility of cancer. I promised I would ask the doctor when I saw her on Friday.

Thursday morning I rang the surgery and they said my blood was showing that something was wrong. I still continued to take a relaxed attitude to all of this. On Friday morning I saw the doctor and she confirmed that there was a problem, but said she was not sure what it was. She was still of the opinion that it could be colic, as she had originally thought. I asked if I could have a CA125 and she said to me: "You don't have ovarian cancer."

I know why she was so convinced that I did not have it. She had received a report from Queen Mary's, Roehampton the previous November telling her that the scan I had was clear. It is not surprising, therefore, that she rejected the idea of ovarian cancer. What neither of us knew was that the scan had not gone down as far as the ovaries and was, therefore, useless in the detection of ovarian cancer. She told me to come back on Monday and if there were no improvement, she would send me for an Xray.

The ache in my back was becoming intolerable and my tummy was continuing to get bigger. On the Saturday morning I took Alexandra down to a shop in the village that specialised in miniature furniture. She was redecorating the doll's house and wanted a new bedroom suite. It was an effort for me to walk there and back. I was in pain and I was having difficulty breathing. Returning home, I decided to have a lie down.

Rosemary, who had been a godsend up to now in taking Alexandra out when I could not manage it, arrived about three o'clock. She was going to take her to the adventure playground in Holland Park in Kensington and then to tea at one of the local restaurants. Looking at me lying on the bed, her first words were: "Why don't you go to casualty?"

My reaction was - why not? We explained to Vincey and Alexandra what we were doing and both of us set off for Charing Cross Hospital, which is just over Hammersmith Bridge - about fifteen minutes from where I live. I was dreading what I expected to be a long wait. But I was seen within twenty minutes. For the next two hours I just laid in a bed in casualty. They seemed more concerned about my heart than my tummy. After I had been seen by one of the doctors, he said there was nothing wrong with my heart. I said that I was aware of that - it was my tummy that was causing the problem.

I have never attended a casualty department for myself in my life. And here I was, lying on a bed waiting to see what would happen. They had decided to keep me in. I knew I was not well, but I was not expecting this. My tummy was now so big that I looked as if I was nine months pregnant. I could not eat any solid food and I was even having problems getting down my sips of water, which I was now surviving on. As I write this, I am remembering how miserable I was feeling. I did not want to be there, but I seemed to have limited options.

They would not let me use my mobile inside the hospital, so Rosemary agreed to go back to my house and explain to my poor bewildered husband and granddaughter that I had been kept in.

It was difficult to gauge whether they had a shortage of beds or if it was just convenient for me to stay down in a department that was just off casualty. I was there until Monday morning, when I was moved up to the tenth floor. I might just as well have been at home - it would have been better for me. If at all possible, it is a good idea to avoid hospitals at weekends unless it is an absolute emergency. You just lie there.

If I was expecting some sort of diagnosis on Monday, I was sadly disappointed. The only way to describe the situation was shambolic. There was no sense of urgency. It was obvious to a blind man that I was in distress. They knew that I was not eating and was only drinking small amounts. They could see the size of my stomach and knew that it was painful. Basically - my vital organs - kidneys, liver and lungs were all being pushed out by whatever was in my tummy - wind or fluid. All I discovered on Monday was that I was in danger of catching the dreaded hospital superbug because of the grubbiness of the ward - it was dirty and the bathrooms and toilets smelled like sewers.

A doctor and a couple of his sidekicks turned up about eleven o'clock, asked me how I was feeling, said I would have to go for tests and then wandered off. That was the end of Monday except for the usual blood pressure and temperature.

I had been quizzing the nurses all day - what could it be that was causing this and what could be done about it. The general consensus was that if it were fluid, it could be drained, but no one was making any decisions.

Tuesday was not much better. Once again the doctor turned up with a young woman doctor, asked the same questions and was not very forthcoming when I asked him if he had any idea what was causing my tummy problem. He said he would know more after the tests. I was becoming more and more distressed. I could hardly walk because my stomach was so swollen. I waddled everywhere - whether going to the toilet or trying to have a bath. I did, however, make some small progress - I had a scan. This should have identified what was wrong and I suppose it did to a degree - but there was such a mass of what I now know to be fluid that it was not very clear. The radiologist was having difficulty in seeing what was there, but he saw that there were cysts on my ovaries. I can't remember who told me. It could have been the radiologist or one of the doctors. I was still not concerned, just in pain. I had heard of women who had cysts on their ovaries. Nothing ever came of them and they were left.

What was more worrying for me now was that I knew it was fluid in my tummy. Based on my newfound knowledge, I could have ovarian cancer. This was one of the classic symptoms. But what I was finding even more difficult to understand and very worrying was that the fluid was almost certainly packed to the gills with cancer cells and no one seemed in a hurry to remove it from my body.

By Wednesday morning, I was beginning to get angry. As far as I could see, I was just being left there. Nothing was being done and there was no sense of urgency. The doctor supposedly responsible for my treatment was quite happy to turn up everyday and tell me absolutely nothing. I was fast coming to the conclusion that the cleaning lady - whom I saw for five minutes a day as she ran her mop down the centre of the ward every morning - would probably have been more forthcoming on my condition had I consulted her.

I went and saw the staff nurse and told her I was planning to check myself in the private hospital on the fifteenth floor - perhaps there I would get something done. She said there was no need - I was going down for a another scan that afternoon to identify where the best place was to insert the hole needed to drain off the fluid. They were going to do something at last.

To this day I still do not understand why it took so long for this to happen. I mentioned this to one of the cancer nurses at Hammersmith months later and she said that the doctors don't always recognise the symptoms, which is why they don't react with any sense of urgency, but added that there was no reason for not removing the fluid. This I found very scary.

Thursday morning started much like any other morning - but this time there was going to be some action. Or so I thought. My side had been marked the previous day and I was now waiting for the doctors to arrive and get started - apparently it needs two of them. Then I discovered that it would not happen until two o'clock, according to the staff nurse who had organised it.

Pauline rang about twelve o'clock for an update. She was planning on coming up from Hampshire on Friday morning if the fluid had not been removed. I was becoming more agitated. I nearly drove the staff nurse mad - I was down at the nurse's station every half-hour demanding to know if these two doctors were definitely going to turn up and insert the drain. By now I had little faith in anything that was said. I saw another weekend looming with nothing done and I was becoming more and more distressed. I can say in all honesty, I will never go near Charing Cross Hospital again, no matter how ill I am.

At two o'clock a German woman doctor arrives. She is part of the duo. But the other doctor - the one I see every morning - is still missing. He eventually arrives half an hour late. By three o'clock, the tube is inserted and the draining operation begins. I cannot describe the blessed relief of the pressure being taken off my stomach.

By eight o'clock in the evening, I was beginning to feel human again. I can see the fluid pouring into the catheter-like bag that is resting in a frame on the floor and with each drop the pressure is eased and I am beginning to feel good. I still don't want to eat, but I continue to sip water. I now also know - I am ninety-nine per cent sure - that I have ovarian cancer, although it has still not being confirmed by any of the medical staff. I am not that concerned. I've had cancer twice before - what was there to worry about, I ask myself? But I decide to say nothing to my family until it has been confirmed.

Friday morning the young woman doctor who has accompanied the lead doctor - for the want of a better description - arrived about ten o'clock on her own. She said that she was expecting the results of my blood tests in the afternoon and would be back to tell me what they were.

I was in a much better frame of mind. The fluid was continuing to flow out and I could see my tummy physically getting smaller. I could move about with some ease and went for walks down the corridors clutching my fluid bag.

In the late afternoon, she returned. I could see by the expression on her face that she was the bearer of bad news. She said the tests had confirmed that I had ovarian cancer. I remember that I started to cry and she tried to comfort me by saying that there were lots of things that could be done today. I explained that I was not upset because I had cancer, but because of what it would do to my poor, long suffering family - particularly my husband and my daughter - who would take it badly. I was putting them all through the wringer again. She tried to cheer me up by telling me that the one I now called the lead doctor - I never actually saw the consultant who was ultimately responsible for me - had posed the question was I normally so bad-tempered. I have to say I was far from pleased that an Iranian doctor working in the NHS should be more concerned about a patient's temper rather than their illness. I said to her that if he had shown a little more urgency, I might have proved to be better tempered.

She then went on to explain that there was no department at Charing Cross Hospital to treat ovarian cancer and I would have to be transferred to another hospital. I was delighted to hear this - I don't think I would have stayed there anyway. The decision was made that I would go to Queen Charlotte's Hospital in Du Cane Road for my operation and then I would attend the cancer clinic at Hammersmith Hospital, which was considered a centre of excellence. I would be transferred to Queen Charlotte's on Monday. Meantime, I had to stay in hospital until all the fluid had drained off.

With no knowledge of ovarian cancer, I was curious as to what its effects were and, more importantly, what its survival rates were. Both of my previous cancers had been treatable and I have to admit, I was taking the same attitude with this one. I never really thought that I would need radio or chemotherapy. I quizzed the nurses, but they were less than forthcoming. When I pressed them, the only piece of solid information I got was that it depended on the stage it had reached. And as no one seemed to know which stage I was at, it was difficult to judge. I knew the lack of information was not the fault of the nurses - they were not being secretive. It is very difficult for them - they are not really allowed to say too much to patients. Apparently this is the prerogative of the doctor.

I did not realise that the NHS had weekday wards and weekend wards. This I discovered on Saturday morning when a nurse came and told me that I was going down to the seventh floor because the one I was on was closing until Monday morning. My reaction to this was that I could go home instead. I had already been making inquiries. If I were not going to another hospital until Monday, why should I not spend the weekend at home, was my thinking. I was feeling really good. There was also another reason - I was starting to feel hungry and I was longing for an omelette. I don't like hospital food. Whenever I had been in hospital before, I usually survived on sandwiches brought in by my husband. I now wanted to go home and have an omelette for my breakfast and my Sunday lunch.

With all of this in my head, I packed my belongings and a nurse escorted me down to my new home. This was a pleasant enough ward, much bigger than the one I had just left. About twelve o'clock, a young doctor turned up to see how I was and to check the speed of the drain. Apparently if it comes out too fast, your tummy implodes with the resulting problems. The nurses on the new floor were very nice and had told me that if all the fluid had gone by Saturday evening, the doctor would probably agree that I could go home on Sunday morning. My first question to him when he arrived was - can I go home tomorrow for the day? After checking the progress of the fluid, he said that there did not seem to be much left and he would come back later and remove the tube. Once that was done, it would be all right for me to go home in the morning for the day. His words were like music to my ears - I was delighted. He also told me where to find a good supply of books - he saw I was near the end of the current book I was reading - should I need any more. I was not sure if he was telling me that there was a possibility that I would not be going home. I think I was becoming paranoid.

I spent most of Saturday afternoon and evening reading, apart from the time when I had visitors. Late Saturday night, the fluid seemed to have stopped. I was astonished to discover that there had been seven litres of fluid in my stomach - they had measured all of it. No wonder I had been in agony and feeling miserable. My delightful young doctor was back and removed the tube. What a relief - I could now lie on my side and move around with ease. But the best news was that I would have Sunday at home. I would return Sunday evening. On Monday morning I was to have another scan and in the afternoon I would be transferred to Queen Charlotte's, where I would have my operation.

While I was at home I decided to check up on ovarian cancer in my medical book. The comments were mixed. If it were really bad, you had an operation and possibly chemotherapy or radiotherapy. The less aggressive alternative was that you had your ovaries removed. I did not know which applied to me, but I hoped it would be the latter.

I was off again on another of my cancer journeys, but this one would prove to be the most difficult one yet. It had one big question mark over it - would I survive it, not a question I was accustomed to asking.

Chapter 6

Hello Queen Charlotte's

My arrival at Queen Charlotte's, a maternity hospital with a ward dedicated to what they call women's problems, was a very low-key affair. In the late afternoon of Monday, the twenty-fifth of May, I was brought from Charing Cross Hospital in Hammersmith to QCH in Du Cane Road, Hammersmith, by one of those ambulances that look like estate cars, but are cream coloured and have NHS Ambulance Service emblazoned all over them.

There was only the driver and myself. I sat in the back and as we drove through the late afternoon rush-hour traffic, I watched the cars, vans and lorries - all bumper to bumper - as we whizzed along the bus lanes. It had a surreal feel to it - like something out of a Stephen King novel. It was as though it was happening to someone else and I was a spectator.

Twenty minutes later, we pulled up in the front of a newly built hospital and the driver waited for me to get out. Cars were parked everywhere and at every angle - car parking space was obviously at a premium and the cars were squeezed in anywhere a space could be found. I had to ask the driver where the entrance was. Pointing to a door in the side of the building that was not immediately obvious, he said, "See reception," and pulled away. This was the first time I had ever seen this hospital. I'm sure I drove past it many times, but I have no recollection of ever having seen it.

Queen Charlotte's is a bright, airy, pale-bricked building with dark blue paintwork and pale blue tiles. It is less than ten years old.

Attached to the older Hammersmith Hospital building - it is built on to the side of it - it replaced the original and very old Queen Charlotte's Maternity Hospital that was located in Ravenscourt Park before it was closed down. Most of this I saw in a haze. I needed to take a second look later to confirm that my first impression was correct.

Once inside, the woman on the reception desk rang up to the ward and told them I was downstairs. Asking me to take a seat, she said someone would be down soon.

Clutching my case in one hand and my medical file in the other, I went and sat in one of the empty seats to wait. It was now about six o'clock and the reception area was deserted. There was an eerie silence about the place, without the bustle of a busy hospital. About ten minutes later a nurse came down. Her first words were: "Did no one bring you over?" I explained that I was feeling OK and was able to get here on my own without an escort. She did not seem impressed with my reply. Taking my case, we went up in the lift to the second floor and she explained on the way that she would be looking after me all the time I was there.

The second floor was a large self-contained unit that specialised in women's problems, such as wombs, ovaries and periods. You entered it through double doors that are kept locked. Once inside, you are in what is basically a long, wide corridor that I was to become well acquainted with. It had an open plan aspect. On the right were bathrooms, toilets, the kitchen and the nurses' station. On the left were a series of wards, some with six beds, some with four beds and a couple of rooms with only one bed. The nurse guided me down the corridor to what was to become my place of residence for nearly a month. The ward was at the bottom of the corridor, facing the TV room. It was pleasant enough - four beds and a shower room and toilet.

I didn't notice much of this on my arrival, I was still in a daze. The ward was empty and the nurse asked me if there were any particular bed I would prefer? I chose the one beside the door. After all the usual checks - confirm name, address, date of birth, blood pressure taken, temperature checked, questions asked - are you allergic to this are you allergic to that, are you on any medication etc.etc - were completed, I put on my night clothes, got into bed and phoned Vincey.

He had wanted to come to the hospital with me, but I told him it was unnecessary and promised that I would ring him once I was settled in. I was trying desperately to keep down his stress levels - hospitals send them sky high. He was already stressed at the latest cancer debacle and I was terrified that he would have a stroke or a heart attack if he got any more stressed.

Hospitals do not appreciate you using mobile phones for obvious reasons - they interfere with hospital equipment. So they try everything to persuade you to wait until you are either off hospital premises or encourage you to use one of the landlines. It was, therefore, very useful to have a private phone by my bed. Yet I found it puzzling when I saw many of the patients continue to use their mobiles and wondered why they were ignoring the landlines. As it turned out, these people were much more street wise than I was.

The reason was cost. I could not believe the size of my phone bill at home when I saw it months later. Every time my husband, daughter, granddaughter, sisters or friends rang me - they would get a bill for the call - at astronomical rates, much higher than a mobile. The cost of using these phones must have been distressing for anyone trying to survive on state benefits or a small pension.

I mention this now because a pattern soon developed that my husband would ring me twice daily - in the morning and the evening, and sometimes in between despite the fact that he visited every day. We were on the phone for a minimum of ten minutes at a time. It was not that I resented the cost - if that is what they charged who was I to tell them differently. What annoyed me was that there was no information on the cost of the calls, so I was not in a position to make a decision as to whether to use the phones or not. I am not saying that I would have followed the rest of the patients and used my mobile. But I would like to have known.

With Vincey now reassured and promising to see me the next day, I settled back in bed and looked around me. This was my first opportunity to take in my surroundings properly. They were quite pleasant. I could see nothing that might cause a problem. The ward was nicely decorated with matching bed curtains and walls. There were four beds - two on each side and the toilet and the shower in the corner beside the window. Under the window and facing the door was a wash-hand basin. It was quiet, away from the hurly burly of the wards facing the nurse's station. And it seemed less shambolic than Charing Cross Hospital.

There were two reasons I chose Queen Charlotte's. The first was that it came highly recommended. And the second was that it was not difficult for Vincey to travel to by public transport or taxi. He has limited sight and is no longer able to drive. Although Charing Cross is closer, I was pleased that they did not have an oncology department because I was not forced to make a decision between convenience for Vincey and my dislike of the hospital.

Queen Charlotte's was billed as the place to be if you were suffering from ovarian cancer. For not only did you have access to some of the best surgeons that specialised in these type of cancers, but the cancer clinic in Hammersmith Hospital was claimed to be a centre of excellence. Not that any of this was important to me at the time. I had still not realised the true significance of ovarian cancer, how horrendous it was, nor did I realise that it was life threatening. But despite my lack of knowledge surrounding this disease, I was interested in the treatment and how effective the hospital would ultimately prove to be.

For instance, the clinic at Hammersmith had its own blood experts, a dedicated laboratory that turned blood tests around in a couple of hours - that is good, apparently, for the NHS - and nurses who specialised in cancer treatment. I was to understand later the true meaning of these facilities. But for the time being, I was just pleased to be told that some of the country's top consultants practised at the cancer clinic, which I would probably attend later as an outpatient, dependent on the outcome of the operation.

I was told the clinic boasted all the vital back-up services necessary for the efficient and, hopefully, effective treatment of ovarian cancer. Then there was the added bonus that there was regular contact between the resident consultants and the researchers at the Royal Marsden, one of the most famous hospitals in the world for cancer research and testing new cancer drugs. And if that there were not enough, once you had completed your treatment at Hammersmith, you were referred back to Queen Charlotte's for regular check-ups.

This was all very encouraging. If you are going to have treatment for the worst illness you have ever had in your life, it helps to know that those who are treating you are the best at what they do. It also helps that they are all under the same roof - despite being separate hospitals - and the fact that they are with you from start to finish. For some reason that I cannot explain, that old labour party slogan - from the cradle to the grave - came into my head and made me smile.

About an hour later, in what was the middle of the evening visiting hours, a doctor came to see me and said that they would probably be performing the operation on Thursday afternoon - about two o'clock. In the meantime, he explained, I would need to go for some tests and a scan between now and Thursday. I explained that I had already had a scan at Charing Cross. He said: "We like to do our own."

All of this was running through my head, as I lay in bed unable to sleep. I gave up after a couple of hours and went to the TV lounge in search of something to read. Everywhere was quiet and in semi-darkness. The night nurse spotted me coming out of the TV lounge and came to see if there were any problems. She offered me some sleeping pills when I explained that I could not sleep, but I declined and said I would probably fall asleep reading.

Tuesday morning, the nurses were about early doing beds, dishing out medication and the eternal checking of blood pressure and temperatures - a ritual that is performed at least three times a day. The food trolley follows all this activity. If you plan to eat in hospital, the procedure is that you choose in advance the food you want for the next day from a menu that is placed on your bed. If you are new and have not had the opportunity to do this, you get what the previous tenant of the bed had ordered or a sandwich.

I could not eat again. For some reason I was back in my not hungry mode. I thought this had all stopped when the fluid had been removed. But once again, I did not seem to be hungry. I just drank water or lemonade.

A couple of hours later, the gynaecologist visited. I don't remember much of what she said. Somehow, it did not seem relevant, which is probably why I don't remember. Vincey arrived about eleven o'clock and left two hours later. Sometime after he had gone, I was taken by wheelchair across to Hammersmith Hospital - you don't actually leave the building you just traverse a series of corridors and a lift - for a scan and an Xray.

You have to wait for the porter to come to the ward to pick you up. Then you have to wait down in the imaging area for the technicians to do the Xray and the scan. And finally you have to wait for a porter to come back and take you to your ward. There is nothing to do but wait and I hate long waits.

On Wednesday, Vincey arrived about twelve o'clock and left two hours later, promising he would be back tomorrow about eleven o'clock, to see me before I went down to the theatre at two o'clock. Just after he left, Karen Somerfield, the Macmillan nurse, arrived.

I don't remember that much about my initial meeting with her other than that she was very helpful and insisted that if there were anything she could do to help, I was to let her know immediately.

I got to know Karen very well later and my first thoughts about her were more than correct. She proved to be twice as good as I had originally thought. She went through everything with me and said if I needed help with anything - either now or later when I left hospital - she would organise it. She proved to be true to her word.

In the afternoon, Rosemary arrived. We chatted about this and that and she left when I started to fall asleep. I had started to dose off during the day, but then I would be awake all night reading. The anaesthetist arrived about seven o'clock and went through the procedure for the next day, explaining that he would be back tomorrow for the premed. I was scheduled to go down to the operating theatre in the afternoon, he told me.

There was no sign of my old friend *nil by mouth* at the top of my bed. I think this instruction has been phased out. Not that I needed reminding. I didn't want any food. The sum total of my intake was sips of either plain water or barley water.

Once again, I spent most of the night reading, trying not to think about the ordeal that lay ahead. I would have no influence over what happened tomorrow. All I could do was hope that there would be no disasters.

Chapter 7

Operation and dreaded E.coli

The morning of the operation was no different from any other morning - beds made, blood pressure and temperature taken, medication handed out, the breakfast trolley and the lady with the mop - that was the order of things - the everyday routine.

So far as I was concerned, the only difference this morning was that I was having a hysterectomy - the first major operation that I have ever had in my life and one that did not guarantee success. The plan was to cut out as much of the cancer as possible and if there were any left, to blast it out of existence with chemotherapy, a plan I fully endorsed.

I was scheduled to go down to the operating theatre in the afternoon and was trying very hard not to think about it. I was expecting Vincey to arrive just after eleven o'clock, as planned. I needed to see him, even if it were just to say hello. But for some reason that I was unaware of, they brought the time forward and I was taken down three hours early, at eleven o'clock. I did not get an opportunity to ring him and tell him about the change of plans. One minute I am lying in bed staring into space, the next my bed is being turned into a trolley and the anaesthetist is there with his potions and needles and I am on my way into the unknown.

When Vincey arrived and saw that the bed had gone, he did not know what to think. He went off to see one of the nurses to investigate and she explained that I had gone down early, but did not say why. He sat in the ward waiting for my return and after about two or three hours he started to get worried. Why was the operation taking so long? Something must have happened to me, he reasoned.

I knew nothing about any of this until the next day when one of the nurses asked me how my husband was. Seeing my puzzled expression, she explained that he had been very upset the previous day and insisted on seeing me. The only way they could pacify him was by taking him down to the recovery room next to the operating theatre, so that he could see I was still alive. He had convinced himself that because I had been gone for so long that something dreadful had gone wrong with the operation and I was dead. My poor, long-suffering husband had being put through the wringer again.

The thing about operations is that you are totally unaware of all the worry and stress you are causing. It is your family that suffers as they wait to see the outcome. I don't remember seeing Vincey. I don't remember coming back to the ward. I remember nothing. The only recollection I have is of a woman standing at the bottom of my bed who said she was the doctor who had performed the operation and telling me that they had removed everything they could, including the apron, which I had never heard of. Apparently it is a thick protective skin that hangs down like an apron and was needed to protect the stomachs of our ancestors thousands of years ago if they were attacked by wild animals while hunting, but is now no longer needed. My inside had been covered with cancer, she said, and there was still some left. I was still hazy from the anaesthetic and didn't know whether I had dreamt the whole thing. Months later I was able to confirm that it was real.

Next day, when the anaesthetic had worn off and I was fully awake, I started to realise how painful an operation it had been. I had a wound that was about nine inches long and my entire stomach felt red raw. I could barely move without it hurting. Although they were feeding me painkillers, it seemed to make very little difference. I was able to talk a little, but I could hardly hobble to the toilet and I was not able to eat. All I could do was have the odd sip of water.

I had never had a major operation before and I did not know what to expect. I thought it would be painful, but I did not expect to feel so incapacitated. The doctors on their daily rounds seemed pleased with the outcome. Everything had gone according to plan - the operation was a success, they said, despite the fact that they were unable to remove all the cancer - and there was every reason to believe that I would be able to go home in about a week. This was all good news and I was delighted that I would be going home so soon. However, I now had to face the prospect that I would need chemotherapy or some similar type of treatment. This was not one of my usual cancers. This was a new breed that I had never encountered before and I was not very well acquainted with it.

I am generally very active and lying in bed was proving to be a whole new experience that I did not like. For the first few days, I was so exhausted that I just lay there sipping water, sleeping during the day except when I had visitors and reading all night. But by the end of the third day I started to make progress - I was eating small portions of custard, the first solid food since before the operation. Moving around in the bed was still agony - so I tried to stay in the same position for as long as possible and I only got up when absolutely necessary. But I was eating and starting to feel slightly better.

Then, without warning, my temperature shot up and I began to feel dreadful. I stopped eating - the small amount of food that I was managing to get down was now making me sick. I could not take any of my medication - I just brought it straight up again - so a drip was fitted to stop me becoming dehydrated. It was *nil by mouth* - but only because I could keep nothing down. My medication was administered either through the drip or by injection. The doctors continued their daily visits, checking my wound, but saying very little. One day, a very pleasant young Australian man came and took blood from my arm, but did not say why, only that it was needed for testing.

I did not know what was wrong with me and could not understand why I was having what I can only describe as a relapse. The first two days after the operation I was feeling fine, now this. And there seemed to be no explanation.

On the fourth day I was told I had an infection - the blood results had come back - and I was prescribed antibiotics. My temperature continued to stay stubbornly high and any thoughts I had of going home were soon abandoned. I could barely walk and I was neither eating nor drinking. I had assumed that the infection was the result of the operation and no one told me anything different. So I just lay there with my thoughts. I could no longer concentrate on reading, but I kept my mind active planning my sister Pauline's birthday party. It was the one thing that kept me sane.

To understand why I was planning her party it is necessary to go back six months in time, long before I expected to be as ill as I was now. Pauline's birthday falls in December, a cold month, and she had decided that as this was a big one - her sixtieth, it would be celebrated in the summer, six months early and not in Hampshire where she lives, but somewhere warmer, different, even exotic. We had spent weeks discussing a possible venue. Her first thoughts were Dublin - where both of us had been born and where we still had a brother, sister, hundreds of nieces, nephews, cousins and in-laws living. But that idea was abandoned for some reason that I cannot remember. We then looked at the possibility of New York. That would have been ideal but for one reason - Vincey hates flying. I would not get him on an eight-hour flight, no matter how hard I tried. The only reason I get him to fly to Spain is because he will see his daughter, his son-in-law and his beloved grandchildren. But this was supposed to be a family celebration, so we would not go without Vincey even if he wanted us to, so we dropped that idea. We looked briefly at Menorca, in the Balearics, where Jackie has a beach house, but decided against that because she was in the middle of some building alterations.

After much consultation and negotiation, we finally settled on a garden party at my house. Not as exciting as New York, as interesting as Dublin or as relaxing as Menorca, but it was convenient for everyone. I'm sure Pauline would have preferred somewhere a little more exciting, but it was not to be. It was agreed that the party would be held on the last Saturday in July, which we hoped, would prove to be warm. London was ideal for everyone's travel arrangements and Jackie, Gilberto and the children would stay with us while everyone else coming from Dublin would stay in Hampshire with the birthday girl. They would all drive up to my house on the day.

I decided that I would let the children decorate the garden - they would enjoy that. Once they were in London, I planned to take them to one of those shops that sell all those fancy party decorations and they could choose what was needed. The theme, we had all agreed, would be oriental. This was mainly for convenience - there was a good Chinese restaurant close to where I live and we would order the food there and have it delivered. The table would be dressed in red and gold and we would festoon the trees in the garden with brightly-lit lanterns, streamers and balloons. There would be cocktails on the patio and we would eat inside. I went over this in my mind so many times that I started to fancy Chinese food.

Pauline was ringing every day to see how I was and to see if I needed anything. As she was planning to drive up from Hampshire to see me in a couple of days, I asked her if she could bring me some Chinese food. I was convinced that I would be able to eat it. When she arrived, she had so many foil containers that I thought she had brought the entire restaurant menu with her. I ate two spoonfuls of rice and was immediately sick. That was the end of my food fancies for the foreseeable future.

About this time, two things happened that changed my attitude to hospitals in totally opposite directions. It was the first time I had seen so clearly the two sides of the National Health Service - one bad, one good.

The first was that I discovered purely by accident why I had been so ill. I had contracted the E.coli bug. My illness was nothing to do with my operation and everything to do with the hospital. I was horrified and tried to find out how this could have happened, but I was getting no answers. I was too ill to make a fuss and to this day, I do not know how I picked it up. I have had numerous suggestions from both medical staff, visitors - everyone, in fact, seemed have a theory. But the culprit appeared to be the plastic water jugs and glasses they give you. Although they are changed daily, I was told that they are not sterilised, and I had been sipping water continuously from the glass.

What was even more disturbing was that I found out about the bug because of a chance remark by a nurse. The night nurse had forgotten to give me my late night injection and came back thirty minutes later stating: "You need your E.coli medication." I was half-asleep and barely took in what she said. It was not until next morning, when I woke up, that I realised the significance of her statement. I needed to talk to her immediately to confirm that I had not dreamt the whole thing, but she was busy preparing for the arrival of the day shift and I had to wait until she was just going off duty before I was able to quiz her. She did not seem that surprised that I did not know and said it was the reason I was on such heavy-duty medication.

When I told my family about the E.coli, there was a major furore. Pauline, who is the legal beagle of the family, was on the biggest soapbox she could find, threatening the local health authority with so many writs that they would be buried under the weight of them for months to come. She was closely followed by the rest of my family - all determined to make the hospital pay for its negligence. I was almost on my knees - despite the fact that I could not kneel - begging them to leave well alone. There was nothing to be gained by forcing the NHS to spend money on legal battles - much better to invest it in preventing patients from picking up these bugs in the first place. Calm was finally restored.

The second thing that happened was that a lovely Danish nurse decided I needed help if I was to get better. She knew that I was neither eating nor getting any exercise - both essential ingredients if I were to recover. So with this in mind, she called in the services of a dietician and a physiotherapist - both of who came to see me a couple of days later.

The dietician arrived in the morning, armed with a selection of those high-energy fruit drinks, but I could not get them down. I think I tried every variety, but I could never take more than a sip before it was back up again. To this day, I feel sick at the thought of drinking them. We then went through a list of foods that I might manage to eat and which she would order from the kitchens, but with the same result. Finally, we agreed that I would stay sipping my water, but try adding a little barely water to get my stomach used to something different. I could build on that, she explained. A couple of hours later, the physiotherapist arrived. She spent about fifteen minutes going through a series of exercises with me that I could do in bed and said I should try to walk as soon as possible.

It was now the eighth day after my operation and any thoughts that I had about going home were being put further and further back. I could not eat - only take small sips of water. I could barely walk. I still had my stitches and my wound was weeping in places. I was beginning to think that I was going to be in hospital forever - not a pleasant thought. I knew the only way I was going to get my strength back was by exercise - getting out of bed and walking - once, twice, three times a day - or as much as I could manage. But it proved to be easier said than done. My target, taking into account that it was a struggle to walk the five yards from my bed to the toilet, was from my ward to the nurses' station. This was only half the length of the corridor and back, but in my mind it had taken on all the proportions of a marathon. This was very ambitious considering my condition.

My first attempt was far from successful. I probably did about ten yards and I was so exhausted that I crawled back to bed. But it was a start. My problem was that even after the shortest distance, I would have to lie down for at least an hour to recover. But I was determined that I would try to walk down the corridor to the nurses' station and back.

The E.coli had certainly taken its toll. I looked more like a ghost than a human being - I was so fragile I was almost transparent. I had lost nearly three stones in weight and I would not have looked out of place in a concentration camp. I was skin and bones and my face was so white it was difficult to tell the difference between the sheet on the bed and me. If I had any doubts about my ghost-like appearance, they were soon dispelled, judging by the looks on the nurses' faces as I passed them. Out of their mouths came words of encouragement. Out of their eyes came pity. Bent almost double, I could not stand up straight because of my stitches. I looked like someone at least twenty years older as I shuffled up and down the corridor pushing my IV stand. Without it, I would probably have keeled over. My second attempt was marginally better. I hobbled up and down the corridor, hanging on to my stand like a drowning man hangs on to a log, then falling into bed exhausted. I congratulated myself on getting there and back without collapsing. But despite everything, I was improving. Within a couple of days I started to accompany Vincey down the corridor to the door when he was leaving after a visit. I had to stop for rests regularly, but it was a major improvement. Seeing that I was making progress, he decided that the walking was doing me some good and I should try harder. So he suggested a more ambitious target, walking up and down the entire corridor. This was impossible, but I managed half the corridor twice a day. Every morning when he visited, he wanted to know how many times I had walked the previous day.

Although I was still not eating, I was slowly recovering. My stomach was still very sore and they continued to delay removing the stitches. On the eleventh day after the operation I was able to take a shower - previous to that I was washing by the side of my bed. I did not have the strength to even sit down in the shower. It took me nearly three hours to recover, but it was worth it - I cannot describe to you the feeling - it was wonderful. I was glowing - this was the best I had felt in nearly three weeks. When the doctors arrived on their rounds, they were surprised and delighted to see how well I looked. I think they sometimes thought that they had a potential corpse on their hands.

Checking my wound, they said the stitches could not yet be removed and it was unlikely that they would let me out. Day twenty of my stay proved to be the most optimistic yet. The doctors said that I could probably have my stitches removed in a couple of days and I was now ready to be passed over to the care of the cancer consultant from Hammersmith Cancer Clinic, a Doctor Iain MacNeish, who would be along to see me soon. They explained that their part in my possible recovery was over, but one of them would be back to remove the stitches. And the best news of all - if nothing else went wrong, I could go home on Friday, five days from then. I thanked them for all their help and assistance.

I persevered with my daily walks, albeit still very slow, and continued to eat some cornflakes for breakfast. Although I only managed a couple of mouthfuls, it was food and I was keeping it down. This was progress indeed. I had decided that I might be able to eat something at lunchtime and asked for soft sandwiches. But that proved to be a disaster - I only had a couple of mouthfuls and threw the lot up. I continued to try to eat, but every attempt ended in failure. Part of the problem was that I could not burp, despite desperately wanting to. I would eat something - then I would feel the need to burp, but I could not. That was the signal that I would not keep the food down, I would be sick. So for a while I was back to my diluted barely water for lunch and dinner.

I counted the days to seeing the consultant. Once that was over, I knew I would be on my way home. I was terrified that if he delayed his visit, I would have to stay in hospital longer.

Some of my thoughts during this time were a bit hazy, but I remember my first meeting with Dr Iain MacNeish, the cancer consultant, as if it were yesterday. It was a Wednesday morning about eleven thirty, two days before I was due to go home. Suddenly - there he was - this very tall, young man whom I did not recognise standing at the bottom of my bed. I guessed who he was because beside him was Karen Somerfield, the MacMillan nurse. A couple of days previously, Karen had visited me and told me that Iain MacNeish would be along to see me and would explain everything about my future treatment.

Iain proved to be a lovely, straight-speaking Scot. He sat by my bedside in Queen Charlotte's Hospital and patiently explained everything in detail, so that there could be no doubts and no misunderstanding as to what lay ahead for me. On the other side of my bed was Karen. Still barely recovered from the E.coli bug - despite the odd good day - and hardly able to speak, I had only one question for him – what are my chances of survival?

Sympathetic, but direct, he said: "Fifty-fifty."

He then went on to explain that I needed chemotherapy to try to remove the rest of the cancer. He said that although my ovaries had been removed and I'd had a full hysterectomy, the surgeons were unable to remove all the cancer, which had spread to my stomach. I would need a course of six treatments of chemotherapy to try to kill it off. He said that the chemo would be a combination of two drugs, which he hoped would prove to be the most effective in killing it. He then explained that I would probably lose all of my hair after the first chemo treatment and went on to enumerate all the other side effects of the drugs.

He took over thirty minutes to explain everything and was more than willing to answer any questions that I might have, to reassure me that this was the best course of treatment for my particular cancer and to allay my fears.

I could not fault him. He was excellent. I was left in no doubt as to what lay ahead, but I have to admit that I was feeling too ill to take in much of what he said. It was at least two months before I could return to the questions I realised that I wanted answers to.

Before chemo is administered, you have to be measured for it. I found this amusing in a macabre sort of way - at least I was not being measured for my coffin. The test is done in the nuclear medicine department. Many times I had seen the sign for this department in Queen Mary's Hospital, Roehampton. Every time I saw it, I asked myself what nuclear medicine could be. I had visions of isotopes and men in white space suits with their arms buried in glass cases full of radioactive substances. Nothing could be further from the truth, as I was to find out. Karen, who had stayed after Iain MacNeish had left, said that she would try to set up the appointment for as soon as possible so that I would not have to come back to the hospital to have it done. It was just as well that she did, because I was in no fit state to come back and sit in the department for five hours, which is how long it takes.

Nothing moves fast in the NHS and it was not until late on Thursday evening that I was told I would be having the test done on Friday morning, the day I was due to go home. It was also when I found out that my daughter was arriving from Madrid. When Vincey rang me on Thursday evening, he said that our daughter was en-route to Heathrow as we spoke. She was on the last London-bound flight from Madrid and would arrive home about midnight. I had tried to dissuade her from coming to London - it was more important to me that she stay with the children, but she had decided that she wanted to be in London, particularly as I was going to be home.

I was awake earlier than usual on Friday morning - probably because I was so excited. I had been in this hospital for over three weeks. Today was a red-letter day for me - for not only was I going to see my daughter, but I was going home as well. I packed as much as I could - but I had to wait for Vincey who was bringing in another bag. It is amazing the amount of gear that you can amass in hospital.

When the food trolley arrived, I had half a bowl of cornflakes for my breakfast, but they were threatening to come up again, so I sat on the side of the bed sipping water and trying to settle my stomach. About ten o'clock a porter with a wheelchair arrived to collect me and take me to the nuclear medicine department. Once there, I was parked outside and told to wait - someone would come and get me.

Thirty minutes later I was wheeled into a room and an Asian doctor took a blood sample and then inserted some coloured dye into my arm. The dye, he explained, would be used to measure how strong my kidneys were. From that they would be able to tell the amount of chemo that my body could take. He said that a doctor would come and take blood from my arm in three hours time and again in six hours. After that I was free to go home. According to my calculations, that meant about seven o'clock that evening. Twenty minutes later I was back on the ward and my husband and daughter were sitting by the bed waiting for me.

I shall never forget as long as I live the shocked expression on my daughter's face. She had never seen me ill in her entire life and now here she was seeing a frail, little old lady whom she hardly recognised. I had changed so much that she was having difficulty recognising me. She tried to cover it up by moving behind the wheelchair, but I could see what she was thinking. This is not my mum, this is someone with a passing resemblance to her. I wanted to hug her and tell her everything was all right, but I did not have the energy. It was all I could do to crawl into bed. The hour and a half of continuous sitting up had sapped my strength beyond anything I could endure and all I could do was lie down. Even talking was an effort.

Seeing I was in no condition for visitors - all I wanted to do was sleep - they sat beside the bed silently watching me. About thirty minutes later they left, my husband promising that he would be back about six thirty to pick me up. I spent the rest of the day lying in bed trying to get my strength back for the journey ahead - going home.

I started to feel slightly better and about four o'clock I finished the rest of my packing. I then had a sleep for about an hour. Not long after I woke, the staff nurse came to tell me that my medication would be up from the dispensary soon and that they had contacted my GP to arrange for a district nurse to change the dressing of my wound daily. In what seemed like no time Vincey had arrived and I started to get dressed. This took me ages - I could hardly bend down and abandoned the idea of putting socks on, despite offers from my husband and the nurse. A taxi was called and I was finally on my way with enough pills and bottles to start my own chemist's shop. The nurses walked with me to the end of the corridor, all making jokes about how much I would miss it and waved me goodbye. Although I had been walking up and down the corridor for weeks, by the time I reached the taxi, I was exhausted again.

If I thought that my journey to Queen Charlotte's Hospital nearly a month before was surreal, my journey home was even more so. Everything seemed to be different, yet I don't know why. I had arrived in the rush hour traffic and I was going home in it. Even my house looked different. I had not realised that my walking in the hospital had all been on the same level ground - there were no steps. It was a struggle to walk up the pathway to the front door and I was surprised that I could hardly get my foot over the doorstep. I collapsed on to the sofa in the sitting room and stayed there for the next two hours. Getting up the stairs to bed would have to wait. I was not in as good shape as I had thought.

Chapter 8

Home at last

My so called week in hospital - that was how long I was told it would take for me to recover from the operation - had turned into nearly a month. I have to admit that I was beginning to wonder while I was there if I would ever see my home again. I knew I was being a bit of a drama queen thinking like this, but it crossed my mind more than once. Now I was home and I was delighted, despite the time it was taking me to get up and down the stairs. Vincey and Jackie wanted to put a bed in the sitting room, but I was not keen on that idea. I preferred the stairs to that option. I was taking about fifteen minuets to get up the stairs and about ten minutes to get down. I had to sit down after every step and rest. But I needed the stairs - they would chart my recovery. They would be my marker as to whether I was getting better or not. I also needed to come down at mealtimes, I spent most of my time in bed, sometimes just lying there other times reading. By getting out of bed three times a day and going down stairs, I was trying to bring some normality back into my life. I could not eat, but I could sit at the table for a short while and pretend I was having my meals. Eventually, I tried to eat or drink something three times a day. I would try a couple of spoons of cornflakes in the morning. At lunchtime it was usually a slice of toast, which I sometimes managed to eat, but mostly failed. And in the evenings I would have a drink of lemonade. I know it was not a lot, but it was at least a start.

But despite my eating and walking problems, I was delighted to be home. The great part of all this was that I was with my husband, my daughter and my granddaughter. I knew I still had a long journey ahead, but for the present I was happy to enjoy things as they were.

Jackie stayed for two weeks and helped her father where she could. He was reluctant to have any strangers in the house helping with the cleaning and cooking and insisted on struggling with it himself. I was sad when my daughter and granddaughter returned to Madrid. Alexandra had been with us for quite a while. When I was in hospital she would ring me and say goodnight before she went to bed. And when I was at home, she would come and sit on the bed in case I wanted to have a chat. I was so sorry that she had to see me in such bad shape.

But it was my poor, struggling husband who was my biggest concern during this time. At sixty-eight years of age, he was far too old and in too poor health to be looking after me. But he was there for me every hour of every day - dogged in his determination to care for me. I was terrified that he would overdo things and have a heart attack or a stroke. I did not want to lose the man who was so much a part of my life that I could not contemplate it without him. To understand my concern, it is necessary to look at his health problems.

Fifteen years ago Vincey had a triple bypass. Now he suffers from angina, has a very particular type of rheumatism that he manages to control with medication; has diabetes and major eyesight problems. He is completely blind in one eye and has less than twenty five per cent sight in the other eye. This is probably the one disability that he hates most because it inhibits everything that he does. Yet despite all of these problems, he never complained once. My caring, volatile husband somehow managed to look after me as best he could. He struggled with the shopping, the cooking and the housework. Before I became ill, we would drive either to the nearest Sainsbury's in Chiswick or the even closer Tesco's in Brook Green early on Saturday mornings and do our weekly shopping. Now he had to shop daily and carry it home, bit by bit.

The most important issue now so far as I was concerned was how to reduce the pressure on Vincey. Apart from housework and shopping, he had to keep answering the phone, which rang constantly. I know that the family had to be kept informed, but we had to find a new system that would reduce the pressure.

Pauline, who lives in Hampshire, rang daily. Frances or her husband Joe, who both live in Dublin, rang daily. My brother Pierce, who also lives in Dublin, was on the phone at least four times a week. Add to this nieces and nephews and it is easy to see why it was a problem. Then there were my two sisters-in-law, Nora and Annette. Both live in the Home Counties and wanted to be kept informed. When Jackie returned to Madrid, she was ringing at least twice daily.

With the family dispersed over such a wide area, the quickest and easiest way to stay in contact was by telephone, but because it was causing such a major problem we had to find a way to handle the calls while at the same time reduce the pressure on Vincey. We eventually came up with a system whereby he would only get three telephone calls a day - one from Jacqueline, one from Pauline and a final one from one of his sisters. They would relay the information to everyone else. It was almost like a pyramid. The top of the pyramid was Pauline in Hampshire, and my sister-in-law in Berkshire. They would advise the next level down and so it would continue until everyone was informed. Not that there was much to report.

When I left the hospital I was told that I would get a letter from the Hammersmith Cancer Clinic advising me when my first appointment would be. As Vincey was unable to drive because of his eyesight, they said that I should arrange for transport to take me to and from the clinic for my chemo.

I was home about ten days when the letter arrived. It said that my appointment was booked for eight o'clock on Tuesday morning, the twenty-ninth of June. I was asked to telephone and confirm if this was acceptable and to advise if I needed transport. Vincey telephoned, agreed the appointment and somehow managed to arrange for the ambulance to pick us up.

This was our first experience of a hospital transport department. The one thing that we learned was that they seldom answer their phones.

Although I was continuing to make progress, it was very slow. I could not understand why I needed to stay in bed. I just did not have the energy or strength to do anything else. I was still eating very little - I had now progressed to having very milky porridge for my breakfast - but nothing for lunch or dinner. I had stopped eating my toast and I was still on lemonade for dinner. That seemed to fill me up for the day. Vincey was becoming more and more concerned and frustrated at my lack of appetite, but there was little I could do. I was just not hungry. When I first came home, I was on medication for a week and I had thought that once it was completed, I would start to eat again and feel better. But it made very little difference. I was still weak and I did not even have the energy to walk around the garden. My stomach was still very sore and hurt when I walked, although the wound had since healed.

For the next couple of weeks we just carried on with the same old routine - my eating was improving gradually, I was walking up and down the garden twice a day. The rest of the time I spent reading or sleeping. One day merged into the next until I could hardly tell what day of the week it was. I had no interest in watching TV, listening to the radio or even reading newspapers. My days consisted of crawling down the stairs for breakfast, lying on the settee for about an hour to get my strength back and crawling back up them again. This was repeated three times a day. I had no interest in seeing anyone or talking to anyone. My entire life was lived through Vincey. He told me what everyone was saying or doing. I would just lie there and listen to him.

Equally, I gave no thought to what lay ahead. I was still too ill to be concerned. I had never had chemotherapy before and I did not know what to expect. I knew nothing about the drugs used in chemotherapy. I did not know their names, how they were administered or even what damage they could do to your body.

All I knew was that in my mind chemotherapy was a horror drug, one that you could easily have nightmares about. This was based on some of the stories I had heard about women who were on chemotherapy and some of the information in the leaflets that we had been given. It seemed to me that the cure could be worse that the disease. The only difference - if you have chemotherapy, the end result could be life. Without it, you were dead.

I now faced the prospect of chemotherapy for the next five months and I was not looking forward to it. I had never been so ill for such a long period in my life before and all I could see were endless doctors, nurses, hospitals - nothing else. But I told my self that at the end of it I would know which part of the fifty-fifty I had achieved. I decided there was nothing to be gained by dwelling on the downside and would take each day as it came. But I was still apprehensive about the treatment, no matter how much I tried to push it out of my mind. I had prepared myself mentally for the loss of my hair - it would grow back again - but I was not sure how I would cope with everything else.

My life was being turned into a diary of hospital visits. In the past I'd had tests, consultations with doctors, day care surgery and even a couple of old fashioned operations. True, all of these combined only amounted to five or six visits a year, of which two were for annual check-ups. But now I was looking at wall to wall appointments that seemed to go on forever - more than I had ever envisaged in my life before. More than I wanted. But what was the alternative? No treatment! That meant no life.

Tomorrow I start my first chemo treatment and I am not looking forward to it. I have not been able to prepare myself and I am wishing that tomorrow may never come.

Chapter 9

First chemo

I don't know where the night went. It is now Tuesday morning and I am up at the crack of dawn. I need the time to get dressed and to crawl down the stairs, so I have to be up extra early. I eat my breakfast slightly faster than usual. The hospital transport department had told Vincey that they could not guarantee what time the ambulance would arrive - it could be earlier than needed. Vincey is coming with me - I don't think I could manage on my own. I am still too weak and sitting up for any length of time usually results in terrible pains in my tummy and aches in my back and lungs. I cannot get comfortable, probably one of the reasons why I spent such a lot of time lying down in bed. I am also puzzled as to why I am taking so long to recover - I am usually over any illness very quickly. This one is dragging on and on and is proving to be the exception to the rule.

We get to the clinic, which is buried at the back of Hammersmith Hospital and almost adjacent to Wormwood Scrubs Prison, far too early. My appointment is for eight o'clock, but the ambulance has come early. It is only seven fifteen and everything is closed.

My first impression is that I have walked into a Kew Gardens conservatory. There is greenery everywhere. It is nothing like a clinic, but very pleasant. There is this very big tree in the middle of the large reception area - directly under a tiered-glass roof that seems to reach to the sky. There are high back armchairs set in a square and all positioned around the tree. They look like chairs for spectators with everyone there to watch the tree grow. On each corner are smaller trees. There is a small café on the right-hand side for coffee and pastries. And to the left as you enter is the reception - now closed. To the left of the reception desk and slightly behind it is the treatment room. In another section of the reception, but further into the room, there is a replica of the trees and the armchairs. This is obviously a very busy clinic, with so much seating.

We might have been early, but we are not the first to arrive. There is another couple sitting across from us and what drew my attention to them is that the young woman has a very odd, white pallor - like nothing that I have seen before - and her head is covered entirely in a soft, pull on hat. I suspect that she is having chemo. I do not realise at the time that this is the uniform of the chemo patient.

My attitude when I left home this morning had been - I have been down this road before - appointments, doctors, waiting - so I know what to expect. But it is nothing like before. Somehow this is different and I don't know why. It is only after my third chemo that I realise I have been an innocent abroad, totally unaware of what lay ahead, and believing everything I am told. This is not a criticism, but a statement of how I felt at the beginning of the treatment and how my attitude changed as it progressed. The people involved - doctors, nurses and administrative staff did not change. I was the one who changed. I saw things through less innocent eyes than previously. I was now more knowing and I responded differently. I suppose I had become chemo-wise. But I did not know any of this on my first visit.

With no one around to ask what the procedure was - we just sat there and waited until someone arrived. I made myself as comfortable as possible and about half an hour later, nurses started to drift in followed soon after by the receptionist. Vincey went to see her and a while later a nurse came out of what I came to know as the chemo room and called my name.

I have never been anywhere near a place dedicated to chemotherapy treatment and I did not know what to expect. But it proves to be nothing special, as I run my eyes around the oblong room - taking in the desk, computer and filing cabinets at the one end and three or four beds at the other end. Windows run all along the top of one wall with a view out to another building. There are lots of blue plastic armchairs - the type that have raised footrests - and it all has a slightly down at heel look with scuffed walls and skirting boards. I suppose, as no one is there to admire the décor, it does not matter what it looks like. But I expected something different, something more appealing. This is the room where the nightmares begin; where the bodies are filled with poison in the hope that it will save them; where dreams of a cure can so easily be shattered, yet it all looks so ordinary. Beside each chair is an IV stand - used to hang the chemo bags on. Next to that is a meter - this is for tracking the speed of the chemo entering the body. Every chair has a pillow in a white case.

The nurse who called me in checks my name off a list and introduces herself. Her name is Jean, she tells me, and she will be looking after me throughout my treatment. If I have any problems with the treatment or I need information, she is there to help, she adds. In her mid-twenties, I pick up on her Australian accent immediately. She has a lovely, easy-going smile and a pleasant manner. Pointing to one of the armchairs, she tells me to take a seat and disappears into a small room. Five minutes later she is back with a tray containing a needle, cotton wool and other bits and pieces. She explains that she needs to take blood, which will be sent to the laboratory for analysis. The result of the blood test will be the deciding factor in whether I am given my chemo or not. As she is inserting the needle into my vein, she explains that it is called a cannula or a line - a needle big enough to drip the chemo through. Once the needle is in, it is closed off. Later, when I get my chemo, the plug will be removed and it will be attached to a tube and the other end attached to the chemo bag and switched on. Sometimes the needle can be hard to get into the veins. I'm sure my veins developed an early warning system about needles.

During the months that followed, the minute the tray arrived, my veins went on red alert and hid. It could take ages to find one. But I did not suffer as much as some women who became so distressed that they ended up in tears - all part of the chemo experience. They can also attach what they call fixed lines - these are narrow tubes inserted into your chest. While they avoid the problem of finding veins - they stay in position until you have completed all of your treatments, which can be many, many months - the big drawback is they cause infections. When they are not in use, they are plugged, not unlike what a plumber does to stop the flow of water out of a pipe when fixing it.

With my blood taken, labelled and en-route to the laboratory, Jean sits with me for about fifteen minutes and explains the procedures. I am the new kid on the block and I need to be initiated. The chemo, Jean explains, will be fed into my body through the vein in my arm and as I am on the top dose, it will probably take between four and five hours. But before any of this can happen, I need steroids - these are necessary before any chemo is administered. She hands me a bundle of leaflets on the side effects of chemo to study at my leisure. I don't like to tell her that I have already been immersed in the horrors of the drug and what it can do to a perfectly normal body that is unlucky enough to have some cells that should not be there. Karen had giving me all the information before I left the hospital and Vincey had studied it in detail, providing me with daily lessons on my future as a chemo patient. But I took the leaflets in case there was any additional information. When she was sure that I understood everything, she fitted a bag of liquid steroids to the IV stand and turned it on - pumping the drug into my arm. Once the bag was empty, she said I should wait in the main reception area for the consultant - Iain Mac Neish - to call me.

The clinic is now starting to fill up. When I go back and sit with Vincey, there are at least another dozen or so women, most of them with the same odd pallor and covered heads. Many were waiting for their bloods to be done, I guessed, because I saw some of them later in the chemo room hooked up to the drip.

We had to wait about an hour - my time recollections are a bit hazy - and then I am called into Iain Mac Neish's office. Standing next to him, I realise he is much taller than I remember when I saw him at Queen Charlotte's. But he is still my matter of fact, say it as it is consultant, a trait I appreciate. Later, as I get to know him better, he becomes my lovely, over-worked consultant. Sometimes, the clinics are so busy that it was not unusual for me to see him having his lunch on the hoof as he sped between the reception area, chemo room and his office.

For now, however, he is the doctor that I will see regularly, far more often than I would want to, given the choice. But it is nothing personal. I am just starting to suffer from doctor fatigue. Although he is very direct in his manner, he is also very patient and kind and shows concern when he asks me how I am progressing. I explain that I am concerned at my slow recovery from the operation. My stomach is still very painful and I have an almost permanent backache. But other than that, I am beginning to feel a little human again, I say.

This generates a smile - he has a nice quirky sense of humour and his response is - "You are recovering from major surgery, not a head cold, and your recuperative powers may take a little longer than usual."

When I think back to those early days and my attitude to recovery, I smile at how naive I was.

He then goes through everything again with Vincey and me - explaining in detail where the cancer is - two lumps in my stomach - which he hopes the chemo will be successful in killing. Vincey quizzes him on the success rate of the drugs and wants to know how they have affected other people. Not an easy question to answer - everyone is different.

Iain then shows us on his computer screen the results of the kidney test done by the nuclear medicine department the day I left hospital. He tells me I have exceptionally strong kidneys for my age. For some reason I ask him if the same is true of my liver, but that apparently is average for my age. Good kidneys are an asset when you have to have chemo, I am told. I have to say most of this went over my head - I did not understand the significance of the numbers - but I was to learn their meaning fast in the months ahead.

My knowledge of chemotherapy drugs was, until then, non-existent. I vaguely remembered reading something about combination drugs, but that was it. Iain had already told me in hospital that the plan was for a combination of two drugs - Carboplatin and Paclitaxel, or Taxol as the latter is generally called. These drugs are specifically targeted at ovarian and lung cancers. The mix, one a nasty drug with bad side effects - the other less toxic - is powerful and together could prove to be my best chance of recovery, he tells me again. I did not know at the time that this was now a tried and tested treatment - the result of research by an American doctor some years previously, who claimed that the combination was more effective than a single drug. But most of this I was to find out later, during my treatment.

Chemo is poison and is only issued on a doctor's prescription and then, only after the doctor has checked your blood count to see if you are up to having the drug. If your blood count is not correct, they won't give it to you. Today, however, everything is fine. My Hb count is 9.9, my WBC is 3.59 and my platelets - which I am to become well acquainted with - is 577. This is all very good. Iain writes the prescription and asks me to give it to Jean, who will organise the chemo from the dispensary. Once again I am waiting out in the main reception area, which is becoming even more crowded. It can take a while for the dispensary to organise the chemo and I am beginning to feel very tired - my back and my stomach are really hurting and I would give anything to be able to lie down. About an hour later - I am losing track of time - the chemo has arrived and Jean calls me back into the treatment room. Vincey can see that I am suffering and he asks Jean if I can lie down. She takes me to one of the beds and organises the stand and the chemo. As I already have my cannula fitted, I lie on the bed and for the next four hours I am hooked up to the drip as the chemo seeps into my veins. Vincey sits beside me to keep me company. I want him to go home; there is no point in both of us suffering, I tell him, but he refuses.

At five o'clock the final drops of the third bag of chemo are emptying into my arm. The tracking machine starts to beep - the bag is empty. Jean comes over, hands encased in plastic gloves and carrying the yellow nuclear waste bucket with the scull and cross bones on it. Everything is removed and carefully pushed through the hole in the bucket. I can now go home. Clutching my bag of medication - a pill for almost everything and with my next appointment made - Tuesday, three weeks from today, Vincey and I head for the transport department. We have been in the clinic for nearly ten hours and both of us are mentally and physically exhausted. We cannot wait to get home.

It is my first visit and already I am fed up with it. Everything has taken so long. There is so much waiting around. I cannot imagine what I am going to feel like at the end of it all. But I feel guilty thinking like this. Somehow it seems ungrateful. They are trying to help me and all I can think about is myself. I should be more appreciative. So I settle for a string of wishes: I wish that I were at home: I wish that there were a better system, like a chemo pill, for example. But most of all I wish that I did not have to be here, a vain wish, I know. No chemo, no life.

Yesterday was exhausting. But today I feel good and I seem to have some energy, although I cannot move too much because of the soreness of my stomach. I think part of the reason for my feel good factor is the steroids. That is what Vincey said. You have to take them before and after the chemo treatment. I took some last night and another two this morning.

I am downstairs when Claire the district nurse arrives. She knew I was having my chemo yesterday and said she would pop in to see how I was. We are in the sitting room, sitting close to the patio doors, which are open. It is a lovely day and I am feeling the best I have in months. It is good to be alive. For the next ten minutes we chat, mainly about how I am feeling and the effects of the chemo. I tell her that if this is how I am going to react to chemo, I will be better in no time. After she leaves, I lie on the settee for a while but I have to go back to bed because my back has started to hurt. I will come down again for lunch.

I stay in bed for most of the afternoon reading and dozing, but I am still feeling good. Vincey is very pleased and passing on the good news to everyone who telephones and even making a few calls himself. I have not had the usual side effects - I have not being sick and I have eaten three meals today. This is all very positive.

In the early hours of Thursday morning, I have to get up to use the toilet. My joints feel stiff and I am having difficulty walking. I wonder what it can be, but back in bed I am soon asleep again and think no more of it. Later in the morning, I go downstairs for breakfast, but it takes me ages. I literally go down the stairs one at a time on my bottom. I am aching everywhere - from the back of my neck all the way down to my ankles, all my joints feel sore and I feel as if I have a temperature. We had been told by the clinic that if my temperature goes above a certain level, I am to come back to the hospital immediately. It could mean that I am allergic to chemo and my body is rejecting it.

Vincey had made me some toast, but I could not touch it, the though of eating makes me feel sick. Vincey studies the leaflets and tells me that this is likely to happen and that we need to get a prescription from the doctor. We decide that I should ring the clinic and confirm all this. Jean is not there, but another nurse explains everything. She says that I need a prescription for anti-inflammatory pills, which will ease the worst of the aches and pains. It would seem I am suffering from inflamed joints. I ring the doctor and it is arranged that Vincey will go and pick up a prescription. He is reluctant to leave me and wants to ring Rosemary to come and sit with me, but I manage to convince him that it is unnecessary. Thirty minutes later he is back and I start taking the required dose. By the afternoon I am feeling much worse and I have to keep getting up to go to the toilet. I thought I was getting a urine infection, which must be the result of the chemo. Claire, the district nurse, had already alerted me to the possibility of urine infections. Apparently, my bladder is still weak from the E.coli bug, which is why I am liable to get the infection. By evening, I am feeling really sick and I have to wrap myself in towels to soak up the volume of urine leaving my body because I am exhausted at trying to keep getting out of bed. Vincey wants me to go back to the hospital, but I see little point. It is the chemo, I reason, and I had been told that it makes some people really ill. I am obviously one of those.

For the next three days I just lie in bed and tried to avoid moving as much as possible. The aches in my joints make me feel as if I have a severe dose of the flu. I cannot eat. I cannot sleep. I am having difficulty drinking, despite the fact that I am supposed to consume at least two litres a day to flush the chemo out of my kidneys. But worse of all, my urine problem seems to be getting worse. I have to pad myself with three big bath towels in an attempt to stem the flow. Vincey is becoming more and more agitated, but I tell him that there is nothing that the hospital can do - they would just tell us to carry on with the same. The truth is I just do not want to see any more doctors, nurses or hospitals if I can possibly help it.

As I lie in bed, my thoughts drift to how I am going to cope with five more treatments if this is how it will affect me. I can't say anything to Vincey because it will upset him and he will ring Jackie and my sisters and tell them what I am saying. This will cause major trauma, so I keep my thoughts to myself. But the cure is proving to be worse than the disease and I am thinking that death has to be preferable to this.

By Tuesday I have perked up a little - mainly because I am no longer pouring water like a Niagara Falls. I ring the doctor to tell him how I am getting on with the anti-inflammatory tablets. He had specifically asked Vincey to get me to ring him and tell him how the tablets were working. Once I had gone through everything about the tablets, I ask him if it is normal to get such a bad urine infection from chemo. He said no and suggests that I ask Vincey to take a urine sample down to the surgery as soon as possible. Once again he is reluctant to leave me, but is finally convinced that it is more important to get the test done than worry about me. I promise to stay in bed while he has gone.

I cannot believe the change that has taken place in just a week. Last Wednesday I felt great. Today, I feel like a wreck. I can't sleep. I can't eat. I am even having difficulty getting liquids down. My joints are still aching, despite the tablets, and it has become agony to walk. The balls of my feet are really sore and my toes are going numb. I spend most of my time lying in bed. But the good news is I still have all of my hair. I was expecting it to be gone by now. A few strands came out when I brushed it, but nothing more. I have to keep finding reasons to be cheerful.

On Thursday afternoon, my doctor rings. I am starting to feel a little better, so I am downstairs lying on the settee. She tells me I have a bad urine infection and I need a course of antibiotics. Could my husband go down to the surgery and pick up a prescription? Vincey says he will go straight away. If this continues, he will be forging a path to the surgery.

The antibiotics have cleared up the infection and I am starting to return to normal. Although I am not eating properly, I have a couple of spoonfuls of cornflakes for breakfast, a boiled egg for lunch and a tiny portion of vegetables for dinner. I eat the same every day.

Unfortunately, I am losing weight again. The small gains I made after I came home from hospital have gone.

For the next ten days or so, I try to eat as much as possible to build up my strength for my next chemo. But it is proving to be a problem. I can only eat tiny portions - I just don't feel hungry. And I have started to get fancies. I want a sausage roll, yet it is years since I have eaten one. This is reducing my food intake even further because I have stopped eating my usual diet. My feet are improving and I can walk a little better, but my toes are still numb. I have started to get cramp in my legs and feet. I am beginning to wonder what is coming next. If this is the cure, I think I prefer the disease.

In the following days, I try to go for walks in the garden and eat as much as possible. I am not very successful, but each day I am feeling a bit better than I was two weeks ago.

I am due for my next chemo tomorrow and I am dreading it. I don't think that I can endure another three weeks of the same again. I can tell by Vincey's attitude to me that he suspects what I am thinking. He is being very positive - it will soon be over, he is telling me, and you will be better. He tries to cheer me up by telling me once I am a little better we'll be able to go to Madrid or even Menorca, if we wish. But I don't believe him.

Chapter 10

Fighting to survive

On Tuesday morning, the ambulance arrives on time and we get to the clinic just before eight. I go straight into the chemo room and Jean, who is already there, does my bloods. Vincey tells her that I cannot sit up for long and she arranges for me to have one of the beds. I lie there for about an hour, perhaps longer, and then Iain comes through and calls me into his office. I relate in detail the whole sorry saga, telling him how ill I have been and how I never expected anything on this scale. The last time I saw him, three weeks ago, he had told me that it was not unusual for women to continue working while getting chemo. I am staggered at this piece of information. How could they? They must be superwomen. I can hardly stand upright, let alone go to work. I can't even look after myself, I am completely useless. I am beginning to wonder if I am becoming unhinged and I ask him if chemo has an adverse affect on the brain?

He checks my bloods and says that I can have my second chemo treatment today, but there is a question mark over what will happen in the future. He does not like what has happened to me and suddenly he is developing reservations about future treatments. But I don't like this, I am like a drug addict. I want my chemo today and the next time and the time after that - I want to complete the course as quickly as possible. I don't want it reduced. I don't want it delayed. I don't want any changes to it at all. If it's reduced, I tell myself, I will have only one drug. The "nasty" one will be dropped, but that is the one that is supposed to be the most effective.

Iain explains that it represents only ten per cent of the mix, but if it were not so important, why give it to me in the first place? I am not happy about this and I tell him as much. I need the two drugs if the treatment is to be successful. He says that he cannot have his patients suffering like this, but I think what he also means is that he cannot have his patients looking like me. I am giving an Oscar performance of the living dead. I only have to look in the mirror to know that. The face that looks back at me is barely recognisable as my own. But I am determined to carry on with both drugs, if possible, and tell him I don't mind feeling bad. He is not convinced and says that he will wait to see how I am after this treatment before he decides.

Back on the bed, Jean fits the chemo bag and it starts to flow. It won't take so long this time because I took my steroids last night and again this morning and I am only having chemo today. Vincey went home once my bloods had been done. It was hard work convincing him that it was not necessary for him to stay. It really exhausts him sitting there all day. I promised that I would ring him when I knew I was getting close to the end of the treatment and he could come straight over. It takes him about thirty minutes by public transport or ten to fifteen minutes by taxi, depending on the traffic.

Around three o'clock I ring. I will be finished soon, I tell him. He is at the hospital in thirty-five minutes and we are home within three-quarters of an hour. No waiting around today. I have had nothing to eat since breakfast and I am feeling peckish. Although Vincey had made me a sandwich before I left home this morning, I didn't eat it. I bought a packet of crisps instead. Steroids seem to have the effect of making me hungry. Vincey decides we will have an early dinner. I cannot believe it - I clean my plate. I take my anti-flammatory tablets. I am working on the assumption that if I take them the same day as the chemo, it might reduce the severity of the aches in my joints.

I feel good, but I know this time that it is the steroids that are buoying me up and there is no guarantee that I will feel good tomorrow. But I am thankful for small mercies - this is becoming my mantra. I am just so pleased when I have a good day.

On Wednesday I continue to feel good and eat breakfast, lunch and dinner, but I am wondering what Thursday will bring. Sure enough, Thursday morning everything is back again with a vengeance. The only exception is the urine infection. It has not returned. I'm off my food again and Vincey is threatening to attach my mouth permanently to the bottle of my latest fad - Lucozade. You have to drink, he keeps telling me. I know I have to drink - the clinic tells me I must consume at least three litres of water a day to flush my kidneys. They would prefer that I drank water, but they don't mind what liquid I consume, so long as I get it down. But everytime I try, I bring it straight back up again. I am back to sleepless nights, so I lie with my earphones plugged in listening to the radio all night between catnaps.

A few days later, I start to get dreadful cramps in my feet. I cannot get rid of them and walk around the bedroom on tiptoe for ages trying to stretch them out. It exhausts me and I flop back on the bed. Every night, for the rest of the week, I am walking up and down the hall for a couple of hours at a time in an effort to get rid of the cramps. I am downstairs in an attempt not to disturb Vincey, but I know he is just lying there awake listening to me. If I stop - usually because I need a rest - he calls out.

With each passing day I am becoming more and more exhausted. The little walks I was having in the garden during the final week of my last chemo have stopped. I no longer have the energy. Vincey is now starting to lose patience with my eating habits and is becoming more and more frustrated. He thinks I have a death wish because I won't eat; I try to explain that it's not that I won't eat. I can't eat. I just bring it up.

I am getting thinner and thinner - so thin, in fact, that I seem to be shrinking. I am starting to look like that concentration camp victim again, only worse, if that were possible. And this time I have the added disadvantage of that awful white skin pallor.

Normally what happens during the chemo cycle is that you have ups and downs. My cycle is spread over three weeks, so I should have at least one good week when I am eating, drinking and getting out of bed. The norm, generally, is that for the first three or four days after the chemo, you don't feel too bad. The next four or five days are usually the worst time and are called the down period. In the final period you feel reasonably OK. That is the theory. And as far as I was concerned that is exactly what it stayed - a theory. The reality is that I have a bad time, a really bad time and then a bad time again. Is it any wonder that I want to get the treatment finished as quickly as possible? I don't generally feel sorry for myself, but I am starting to see the first signs of it and I don't like it. My problem is not with the disease, but with the cure.

By the following Monday, I am feeling so low that I decide to ring Iain and see if he has any suggestions. Iain is not available, but the nurse says she will get him to ring as soon as possible.

I don't know what it feels like to die, but I think I am beginning to find out. I know this sounds melodramatic, but that is what I think is happening to me. I am dying and there is not a thing I can do about it. And in addition to everything else, the balls of my feet are becoming even more painful so that I can barely put them down on the floor. If this continues I won't be able to walk soon. The district nurse, Claire, who visits me once a week, has already told me that if I continue the way I am, they will stop the chemo altogether.

A couple of hours later, Iain rings and I explain what is happening. He tells me to come to the clinic the next morning and to "bring my jimjams" as I may have to stay. Tuesday morning we arrive at the clinic at eleven and go straight into the chemo room. Vincey has to get a wheelchair to take me from the taxi because I am incapable of walking any distance. I go straight to one of the empty beds and lie down. I have been half sitting and half sprawled across him in the taxi for the past fifteen minutes and I can't sit up any longer. Karen, the Macmillan nurse, is there and comes over to say hello. I probably look worse now than the last time she saw me - just before I left hospital. But she is very diplomatic and says nothing. There is no doubt I am going downhill. Soon afterwards Iain arrives. He checks me over, but can find nothing obviously wrong. One of my concerns is that I think my stomach has started to swell and the fluid is back again. But it turns out to be a false alarm. He tells me that I will no longer be getting the same chemo mix. I am going on to a single drug from now on. I feel so ill that I don't care whether I get treatment or not. For a fleeting moment, I think it might be a relief if it were to stop altogether. He says that my body is not up to taking the mix and he can no longer have me in such a frail condition. He also explains that I need to go back to the nuclear medicine department for another kidney test before my next chemo. He thinks the chemo has damaged my kidneys, which is why he is reluctant to continue with the current dosage.

I have to say that I find all this a little puzzling. I know I have never had chemo before and I have no point of reference, but I am not generally such a wimp. I usually survive most of what is thrown at me. But I am obviously not surviving this time. He also tells me I need a blood transfusion. This, I am told, is normal procedure for someone on chemo. I have to come back the following Tuesday to get my blood matched in preparation for the transfusion. Vincey is now openly panicking at my condition. But he is convinced that if I could eat, it would make all the difference. To pacify him, Iain gives me some tablets to settle my stomach. I recognise the name on the prescription immediately - I had taken them to clear up the ulcer they found when I had my operation. I know they won't make any difference, but Vincey is convinced that they will help me to eat and is determined that I will take them. He goes down to the dispensary to collect them and back in the chemo room gets me a cup of water so that I can take one straight away. My stomach decides to reject it, but I keep some of it down.

A taxi is picking us up in ten minutes. Knowing I will have a problem going home, I decide to lie down until it arrives. I am feeling miserable and given half a chance would happily abandon everything to do with hospitals, doctors and chemo. Why couldn't this cancer be like my others - problem free? Yet in the middle of all my gloom, I suddenly decide that things could be worse and I cheer up. There are two reasons for my new-found optimism. One is I don't have to stay in hospital - that is always good. And two, despite the fact that I am on my second chemo, I still have all of my hair. The rest of me may be falling apart, but I still have a good thick head of hair. I know I have lost a little, but nothing that you would notice. This is pure vanity. Here I am, suffering from a life-threatening disease and one of my concerns is whether I am going to lose my hair or not. But it makes me unaccountably happy the longer I can keep it. It is as if there is a perverse battle between my hair and the chemo and I need my hair to win.

Ever since Iain had told me in the hospital that I would lose it all after the first chemo, I had been mentally preparing myself for the Sinead O'Connor look - bald. But, somehow, against the odds, I have retained it and instead I have the Camilla Parker-Bowles look, lots of hair. Once again I am thankful for small mercies. And to add to my pleasure and cheering me up even more, when we got home, I drink a cup of soup. This convinces Vincey that the tablets are working and I am not looking forward to having to complete the pack. He won't believe that the soup was a coincidence and I would have drunk it without taking the tablets.

For the next few days, I try very hard to eat and drink. I know that it is the only way that I am going to recover my strength. But it is proving to be easier said than done. It is even more difficult for my poor, long-suffering husband. I don't know how he is coping with me. He is scared to leave me on my own and the only way I can get him to go out of the house is by getting Rosemary to come and sit with me. Later, as I start to improve, he accepts that I do not need a badysitter, but I have to promise that I won't get out of bed. Instead I lie there clutching my mobile so that I can ring his mobile immediately if I need to and he will come hurrying home. Pauline is trying to be as helpful as possible, but it can be difficult for her because she lives so far away. But she tries to reduce the pressure on Vincey by coming to London once a fortnight and doing a major shop for us. And Rosemary will get anything that we need - all Vincey has to do is give her a ring.

But he still has to contend with me. He is continually worried because I am not eating properly, I am not sleeping and I am continuing to lose weight. Certainly, my sleeping habits have become very erratic. I seem to have turned night into day. I doze on and off during the day and then I am up most of the night. I need to move around to stop the cramp, which has spread from my feet to my legs. For some reason that is not obvious it is worst at night.

I have always loved jigsaws, so when I can't sleep and I can't keep walking because it exhausts me, I start a jigsaw on the dining room table. This particular jigsaw - three thousand wooden backed pieces - I have had for years but never attempted it before because I know it will be difficult. It needs lots of time and concentration. The time I have, but I am not sure I have the concentration or the strength. It is a global map of the world, showing not only all the Continents and countries, but also the trade routes taken by the merchant ships as they navigate the globe. I am probably spending about an hour to two hours a night on it - not every night - only those when I need to go walking. I will sit at the table for about fifteen minutes until my back and stomach become too painful. Then I move to the settee and lie there for about thirty minutes to ease the pain before returning to the jigsaw. I need to improve the amount of time that I sit up.

Pauline's birthday is fast approaching and I am not in great shape. I worry about this because I need to get the food organised and I need to buy her a present. She collects crystal and there has been general agreement that we will each buy her a piece of crystal. I can't go out, so Rosemary gets me a crystal decanter from Harrods. I keep the receipt. If she doesn't like it, she can take it back. The party is next Saturday. Jackie and the children are arriving on Monday and Gilberto on the Friday. I have my blood matching appointment on the Tuesday. Everything is happening at once. With the party only a week away, I manage to ring my favourite patisserie in Kensington Church Street and order a very large strawberry sponge with lashings of cream. Everyone likes sponge and strawberries, so they should be happy. We had decided against a more formal cake.

I usually pick Jackie and the children up from the airport, but not this time. I can barely walk, let along drive. Vincey arranges for a taxi to collect them. They are on a latish flight and the baby, who is four, will probably fall asleep. Travelling with three children, particularly one that is tired, is not much fun.

They are expected about eight o'clock, but don't arrive. When it gets to nine o'clock, I start to panic and get Vincey to ring the taxi company. All they are saying is that the flight has been delayed. Yet when Vincey checks the teletext, the flight has landed. Eventually, they arrive about nine thirty. The baby is half-asleep and everyone goes to bed early. Jackie tells me that she is coming to the hospital with me in the morning.

Next morning, we set off for the clinic about eight thirty. The children are still in bed asleep as we leave. Vincey will prepare their breakfast when they get up. We take about fifty minutes - the traffic is dreadful - bumper to bumper all the way. Wood Lane is closed in one direction, which is causing massive jams. We are in a minicab, so we cannot use the bus lanes. I am still not able to sit up and when we arrive I go straight to the bed and lie down. The journey has been agony. Jean comes and takes my blood for matching, but I have to wait for it to come back, which takes about an hour.

Jackie decides that she wants to talk to Iain and when he stops to say hello, she tells him that she is concerned and would like to go through everything with him. He says he will be back in about fifteen minutes.

He explains what is happening and why, telling Jackie that everyone reacts differently to chemo. Eventually I am told I can go home, but I need to come back Thursday week when the transfusion will be done. I am told that I need three units of blood, which will probably take about five hours to feed through my veins, so I should be prepared for a long day. I am still perplexed about the whole thing. The only reason that I can see for the transfusion is that the chemo has done something else to me besides my kidneys - but I don't know what.

It is lovely having Jackie and the children in the house. Although I am totally lacking in energy and I spend most of the day in bed, the children come and sit with me and we chat. When Jackie takes the girls out shopping - she usually leaves Nicholas behind with us because he gets tired and wants to either go home or be carried. When he gets fed up playing downstairs with his grandfather, he comes up to have a chat with me. I put my knees up so that he can use them as a back rest and he will lie there telling all about what he is learning at school and recites his numbers and letters. He is very amusing and cheers me up no end.

On the Thursday, Jackie takes the children to a shop in Kensington High Street to buy the decorations for the garden. They come back very excited and spend ages telling me in great detail where each piece will go. I notice when I go downstairs that some of the jigsaw has been done. Natalia, my eldest granddaughter, loves jigsaws and she has been adding pieces. We always try to complete one when I am in Madrid. We have until Saturday lunch time to finish it because the table is needed. Jackie, I am delighted to say, has taken charge and is organising everything. I don't know what I would have done were she not here.

The food has been ordered and will be delivered early Saturday evening. The cake is being picked up on Saturday morning. The champagne has already being delivered and Pauline will bring the wine. That just leaves the garden to be decorated and the children will do that on Saturday afternoon. I am becoming excited as everyone gets caught up in the arrangements. Rosemary is coming up early on Saturday morning to help, if needed. My contribution is staying out of the way. For now, however, I am just enjoying having my family around me and I am really excited at the prospect of seeing the rest of them, yet I am also dreading it. I know I am in really bad shape and this will cause upset, but I am trying to be positive. Looks are not everything, I tell myself.

Late Friday evening, Natalia and I fit the last two pieces of the jigsaw and stand back to admire it. It looks great and we are reluctant to break it up. Instead, we decide that we will leave it until tomorrow morning. When it takes ages to complete a jigsaw, it is always hard to take it to pieces again.

Saturday morning dawns bright with clear blue skies. There is always a risk attached to having a garden party in England, even in the middle of summer, so we have a fallback plan. If the weather turns foul, we will switch everything into the house. Everyone is up early as there is quite a lot to do. I have half a slice of toast and a glass of Lucozade for breakfast and go back upstairs out of the way. I would love to be in the thick of things, but I cannot stay upright long enough. I decide to stay in bed all day and try to conserve what little energy I have for tonight. I want to stay up as long as possible and enjoy the company. Between naps I hear all the activity as everyone rushes around putting the final touches to the preparations. The children are particularly excited and I can hear their voices in the garden as they hang the decorations.

The plan is that Pauline, my sister Frances and my brother-in-law Joe will arrive about six thirty. My brother Pierce and his wife were due to arrive late afternoon, but called off at the last minute because of a problem with one of their sons. I am sorry that they will not be there, but they have promised that they will come and see me in the next couple of weeks.

It is soon time for everyone to get dressed and the children come into the bedroom so that I can see their dresses. They look wonderful.

They love dressing up for parties or to go out to dinner. Now it is my turn to get dressed. I put on a silk blouse and a pair of navy trousers with navy shoes. It takes me ages and I might just not have bothered. I look like a scarecrow. I wrap a silk scarf - turban style - around my head. I have noticed that there is more and more hair on my clothes as strands continue to fall out. I have a horror that they might fall into my food as I am eating. The thought makes me feel physically sick, so I am taking no chances and cover my head. I go downstairs, but before I can settle myself on the settee, I have to admire the garden decorations. The children and Vincey have done a wonderful job. It looks great. There are lots of pretty blue, red, green and silver lanterns hanging from the trees and there are balloons everywhere. Halfway down the garden there is a big white and blue plastic strip anchored between two bushes with the words Happy Birthday emblazoned across it. Pauline should be pleased.

Soon the birthday girl arrives and we kiss each other in greeting. She hasn't seen me for a couple of weeks and I can see in her face that she thinks I am getting worse. Behind her are my sister Frances and my brother-in-law Joe. We kiss hello and all go out into the garden. I am sitting at the table chatting when I notice that Frances is at the top of the garden on her own. I go up to her, but she keeps her head turned away. Then I see she is crying. Soon we are both crying. It is six months since I have seen her and she is shocked by my appearance. We sit on the garden seat away from everyone and talk. She is my baby sister and I hate to see her so upset. I try to tell her that my current condition is only temporary, it's all the fault of the chemo, but she is not convinced. Vincey calls us down for the champagne cocktails he has made. After much sniffing and wiping, we join everyone else and toast Pauline. The children can't wait to give Pauline their present and want her to open them all before dinner. So we all go back into the house for the present opening ceremony. She is delighted with her presents, particularly the lovely crystal table decoration bought by the children.

I have been up for less than an hour and I am already starting to fade. The food is being arranged on the table and I am desperately hoping that I can stay up long enough to eat some of it. About ten minutes later we are sitting down and I am having more and more difficulty staying upright. The food looks and smells delicious and I am really looking forward to it. Rosemary is sitting next to me and puts two small spoons of rice and some prawns on my plate. I eat a prawn, really proud of myself when I keep it down. I then eat a spoonful of rice. Gaining confidence, I decide to have some noodles. That is my downfall. I can feel the lot coming up. With a serviette stuffed in my mouth, I try to get up the stairs and into the toilet as quickly as I can. I know I am not going to be eating anymore. I also know that I won't be going downstairs again, so I crawl into bed. I can hear the murmur of voices as I slip into sleep. I know during the evening that there are people in the bedroom, I can hear them moving around, but I make no attempt to talk to them. Then everyone is leaving and they are coming to say goodbye - I feel kisses on my cheek, but I am not registering what is being said to me. It is as if I am in a semi-coma.

Sunday morning I don't feel any better, so I stay in bed. I don't want anything to eat. I just sip the Lucozade by my bed. Jackie takes the children out for the day and Vincey prepares lunch for himself. In the afternoon I ring Pauline to say sorry that I could not stay up for dinner. I could hear her voice cracking, as if she had been crying. I ask her if she is all right. When I say I would like to talk to Frances, she says she is upstairs, but will get her to ring me before she goes back to Dublin on Tuesday.

Monday afternoon Rosemary comes to see me and tells me that everyone was in tears in the car on the way home on Saturday night. The only topic of conversation was how ill I looked and was I going to survive.

Some months later, Pauline told me that everyone was devastated. No one expected me to look as ill as I did. She said that when I walked down the garden to Frances, she saw the entire outline of my spine through my clothes and I was bent almost double like a little old lady. She said that I looked so ill that when they got home they did not go to bed - they were expecting a call from Vincey telling them that I had passed away. This was the first time that she really understood how ill I was. When they were leaving, I had hardly acknowledged them, it was as if I was in a coma. Pauline had always maintained, no matter how ill I was, that I would survive. But that night, she said, she started to doubt her own beliefs. For weeks afterwards, Frances did not stop crying and Joe was giving the task of staying in touch to see how I was. She would not speak to me.

Jackie was going back to Madrid on the Wednesday afternoon and I was going to miss her and the children terribly. Gilberto had already left on the Sunday night.

I knew I had little enough energy to entertain the children and I could certainly not play with them, but it was nice just having them around. If I stayed in bed, I was able to conserve enough energy to have a little chat with them and that was enough. The afternoon that they left, I came down the stairs on my bottom to say goodbye. I had giving up trying to walk, it was too exhausting. But the worst moment came when I was kissing them goodbye. I was not sure I was going to see my daughter or my grandchildren again.

It was about this time that the true realisation of what cancer does to a family became starkly clear to me. I had just had all my family around me and I saw what I was doing to them. I would have given anything to stop the hurt and distress that they were feeling. You might have the cancer, but it is your family that suffers. And there was nothing that I could do to help them or ease their pain.

If ever I needed confirmation of this, I had it as I watched them displaying big smiles when they were with me. They were telling me how great I looked and how I no longer looked quite so sick, yet when I was not there, the question was: how much longer can she last like this? I was at the other end of the spectrum, struggling to disguise how ill I was, not easy when you look more like a scarecrow than the real thing, and the colour of your face is so ghost-like that you would put the fear of God into anyone you bumped into accidentally.

I was trying to stop my family hurting and my family was trying to convince me that I was on the road to recovery. Not surprisingly, no was fooled.

Chapter 11

Overdosed on chemo

I cannot believe what is happening. I have just discovered why I have been so ill and it beggars belief. The results of my latest kidney test are back from the Nuclear Medicine Department and the original numbers used to decide how much chemo I should have were wrong - far too high. Somewhere between the Nuclear Medicine Department, the department at Charing Cross that does the analysis on the test and the figures going to the doctor's screen, a mistake was made. They have been overdosing me on chemo. I have been getting nearly twenty-five percent more than I should. This is scary. Surely there are checks and balances with such a dangerous drug as chemotherapy. My first thought when I heard was how could this have happened. My second thought was to suddenly remember the comments made many years ago by a very close acquaintance, a Professor of Obstetrics. He told me that hospitals were dangerous places and to avoid them if at all possible. At the time, I did not take his comments seriously. Now I know exactly what he means.

My kidneys have been so badly damaged that they can no longer take what would have been the normal amount of chemo that I should be getting. Iain has been forced to reduce the dose dramatically. Now, not only will I just have the one drug, but I will have less of it. The initial dosage of the combined drug should have been around six hundred, not the eight hundred they were giving me, so now I am to receive only four hundred of a single drug to stop it harming my kidneys even further. And just for the record, I didn't have super kidneys either. But now, they are not even average anymore.

But where do I go from here? What have they being doing to me? And more to the point, what are they likely to do in the future? First, I get the E.coli bug, now I have been given too much chemo. Where will it all end? The cure is proving to be far more dangerous to my health than the disease. Yet I don't have a choice - I need to continue with my treatment. I could, I suppose, transfer to another hospital. But what would that achieve. I am now familiar with the way Hammersmith works - if such a thing were possible - and I would have to start all over again with a new hospital. And then there are the doctors and nurses to consider. What have they done wrong? Nothing. All they have tried to do is help me. There is also another important factor to be considered. I don't have the strength or the stomach to go hospital hunting. The choice is made. I am staying - good or bad. I will just have to be more vigilant in the future, although how I can assess when mistakes are made is going to be a problem. The only way around this is to have a consultant as an advisor.

My next appointment is Thursday for my first blood transfusion. I have to be at the hospital before nine o'clock. I am so weak that it takes me over half an hour to get dressed. After donning each garment, I have to lie down. I am exhausted and out of breath. Vincey is coming to the hospital with me. I am in no state to go on my own. We arrive by ambulance in good time and once I am settled in he goes home. I will ring him later. For the next five hours I lie on the bed as the blood is pumped into my veins. I sip my Lucozade, but I don't eat - I am not hungry. When I get home, I go straight to bed. Although I have been lying down all day, I am still exhausted. On Friday morning I am starting to feel slightly better and by the following week I feel human again - the blood is giving me life.

But suddenly the situation changes and by Thursday, strange things are starting to happen. I am sitting at the kitchen table when blood suddenly spurts from my nose. I think I am having a haemorrhage. But I have become so used to odd things happening to me that I just mop it up and put it down to the transfusion. I jokingly tell Vincey

I have a surplus of blood, which is why I am getting rid of some. I don't think he is very amused. A little later, I scratch an itch on the top of my arm and a big blue bruise appears. This is odd indeed. For the next three to four days I continue to get nosebleeds and my arms, legs and body are covered in black and blue bruises. I look as if I have gone fifteen rounds with Mike Tyson.

My third chemo is due the following Tuesday and I decide to wait until then to find out about the blood and the bruising. Pauline has decided that she wants to accompany me. I am pleased for two reasons. I will see my sister again - I have not seen her since the party - and it will give Vincey a rest.

Pauline arrives on Monday night because we have to be at the clinic before eight o'clock and she doesn't want to take a chance on being delayed in traffic if she drives up on Tuesday morning. We get there early and I go and sit on the bed. Jean comes to do my bloods and for some reason that I cannot remember, we have a discussion about my hair. I think it is the fact that I still have a big mop of hair. Jean tells me that there is now a good possibility that I won't lose it. Not everyone does. I ask her why I have been having nosebleeds and she tells me it is probably because my platelets are low. She then asks to see my arms and legs. When she sees the bruising, she says it is unlikely that I will have my chemo today, but it will have to be confirmed by Iain.

An hour later my blood report is back and it confirms what Jean said. My platelets are down so it's no chemo for me today. The needle is removed and a new appointment is made for the following week.

Back home I can't settle. I feel a little hungry, but I can't eat. I want to go to the food department of Marks and Spencer's in Hammersmith and Pauline takes me. We buy lots of salmon - fillet and smoked - in the hope that I will eat some of it as well as other tit-bits that might tempt me. I cannot keep still, despite the fact that it is exhausting me. Then I realise it is the steroids - I have taken twenty tablets since last night. They have wired my blood and I've had no chemo to defuse them.

Later that week, I notice that I am starting to seriously lose my hair. It is coming out in handfuls and falling everywhere. The bedroom floor is covered and Vincey has to keep vacuuming it up. Everytime I go into the kitchen, I have to cover my head. Before I eat, I go out into the garden and spend ages picking the hairs off my blouse or whatever it is I am wearing. I am becoming paranoid about the hairs and I am continuously checking my clothes and everything around me. I am also beginning to think that I have a very contrary body - something I'd never realised before. I am told I will lose my hair and I don't. I am told I will probably keep my hair and it starts to fall out. This becomes the pattern for months to come. Everything I am told, my body does the opposite.

But there is an upbeat aspect to all this. Because I have not had any chemo for nearly six weeks, I am not as weak as I was, probably because I have started to eat small amounts of food. I am also well enough to want to go for a walk, not just up and down the garden, but outside. Vincey and I plan the outing for days. You would think it were a trip around the world that we were organising. I know we won't be able to walk very far, but it will be the first time I have been out - apart from hospital appointments - in months. Finally, the day arrives. It is a lovely, sunny Thursday morning and we are going to walk down part of the road and back. We set out and despite the odd wobbly moment or two, we walk nearly twenty yards down the road before we have to turn back. My stomach feels as if it is being ripped out of my body. I stumble back into the house and flop down on the settee. But I am secretly pleased with myself.

I am still waiting to have my third chemo and as the time for my appointment nears, I decide that I need more information about the disease and its treatment. Because I am feeling a little better, I am starting to take an interest in what is happening to me and I have a need to know more. I did not want to talk to the doctors. I wanted something more informal. The first person that came into my head was Karen, the Macmillan nurse. Karen had told me over and over if I needed any help or assistance I was to ask. So I decided to take advantage of her generous offer. To my way of thinking she would be ideal. She would have all the information that I needed and she would be more than happy to go through everything with me. With this in mind, I make an appointment to see her on my next day at the clinic and we agreed to meet in the chemo room.

By now I am getting fed up with arriving at the clinic only to be told I cannot have my chemo. I am beginning to wonder if it will ever happen, but I am assured that it will. I just need patience. I can already see the problems piling up - the treatment is no longer as straightforward as was originally outlined. My body is becoming more and more sensitive to it and I can see it dragging on for months.

When I arrive at the clinic for the umpteenth Tuesday hoping to have my third chemo, Jean tells me that I will be seeing a new doctor, a Paul Mulholland. I had seen him around the treatment room, but had never spoken to him and knew nothing about him. I later find out that he is a researcher for the charity Cancer Research UK and he spends two days a week at the cancer clinics: Monday at Queen Charlotte's and Tuesday at Hammersmith. The rest of his time is dedicated to research into finding a cure for cancer, which he is convinced will happen, but it will take a while yet.

Meanwhile, as I am waiting for my blood results to come back, I spot Karen and another Macmillan nurse and start to walk towards them. But they both walk straight past me and I stand there wondering what is happening. I call her name with the intention of checking to see if we are having a meeting now or later. She turns around and stares at me with astonishment. "Lyn, I am so sorry. I did not recognise you," she said "You look great. I would not have believed that it was you. The last time I saw you were lying on a bed and could hardly move." I had made some reasonable progress since then. I could sit up and walk.

She then introduced me to her companion, Valerie, a new nurse on the cancer team. The three of us then went to a small room off the clinic where we could talk yet where the nurses could find me when my blood results came back. For the next twenty minutes Karen went through everything with me. This was mostly the information that I had not been interested in when she tried to tell me in hospital.

I now knew that I had been diagnosed at stage three and understood the meaning of this. Had it been stage four, I would not be here having this conversation. She went through the symptoms with me in great detail and I recognised every one. I had suffered heartburn, loose bowels, frequently passing urine, tummy ache, backache and a general feeling of not being very well. I had them all, yet I ignored them because I did not realise that they were harbingers of ovarian cancer. She told me that stage three was challenging for the doctors. Basically, what this means is that you'd better get in all the living you want to do because you are not long for this earth.

The thing I liked about Karen is that while she is sympathetic, she tells you everything, warts and all. I knew none of this. I was too busy just trying to recover to ask any questions except the most basic. She also said that when she had come to visit me in Queen Charlotte's, it was obvious that I was not interested. Although she tried to explain everything, I was not really listening. She then told me about the drugs that were available and said that even if it returned later, all was not lost. I knew very little of this. While I knew that my chances were fifty-fifty, I did not know that even if they managed to rid me of it now, it would be back. Few diagnosed at such a late stage survived more than two years.

This was certainly food for thought and heightened my awareness even more of my treatment. Back in the chemo room I waited for the doctor.

Sometime later Doctor Paul Mulholland called me into his office. He is the opposite of Iain in personality and approach. While Iain is more straightforward, which appeals to me more, Paul takes a more gentle approach and always tries to be positive in assessing my progress. He will highlight the positive rather than the negative. It is probably because of this that our first meeting proved to be so eventful and set the tone for all my future visits.

After the overdose revelation, I have taken to questioning everything that is said and done. Part of the reason for this is that I feel marginally better and can actually think about what is happening to me. The other part is that I have reverted back to my profession - asking questions and expecting answers. I have latched on to the CA125 as an indicator of how my treatment is progressing. It is the only marker I have to judge success or failure. If the treatment is failing to produce results, then I have to ask myself whether there is any point in putting my body through the agonies of having chemotherapy. So as a matter of course, I now ask for my CA125 numbers. I know they are only an indication of how successful the chemo is in attacking the tumours, but there is a certain importance placed on them and their downward spiral. When Paul consulted the screen and saw that I had dropped from one thousand to just over two hundred and fifty in two treatments, he was very impressed.

I explained that the reason for the giant leap downward was probably because I had been overdosed on chemo twice. His first reaction was disbelief. Then, it was that this could not possibly be true, but he was far too polite to actually say that I was lying. I assured him it was true. I told him that as far as I knew, the mistake had been made between the test in the Nuclear Medicine Department and the department that does the analysis in Charing Cross Hospital. Somewhere between those two points the wrong numbers had been used. The only other alternative was that the wrong numbers had been put on the computers used by the doctors. He then asked me how could I trust future treatments? I told him with suspicion. But I had no choice - I had to trust someone. There was little I could do; I knew nothing about dosages or how to measure chemo or even how I would go about securing supplies. I was dependent on them getting it right. I also told him that it had a disastrous effect on my kidneys. I had what now amounted to the equivalent of one kidney. In effect, I had lost the use of fifty per cent of each kidney. Paul tried to be positive about this and said that many people live normal lives with one kidney. I told him I was not impressed with his cavalier attitude to my kidneys. Had I not came with two kidneys in working order? Was it unreasonable to expect to leave with them in the same condition, I asked.

Paul is such a sweetie. Despite my remarks, he is still trying to make me feel better about the situation. He then tells me that I was lucky that I did not get an infection, as it would probably have killed me. I retorted by telling him that not only had I had the worst urine infection in my life, but that I was also surprised I was still alive. I was turning into the patient from hell.

Despite all this, he continued in a calm and reasonable manner to explain that there could be benefits. New trials on dosage were showing positive results. Patients who were able to take higher than normal doses of chemo were achieving better survival rates. I told him that he must have been talking to my husband - that was also his view - zap the little b******* out of existence.

But he was less positive when he assessed my bloods. I could not have my chemo today, my platelets were too low and it was far too dangerous. We laughed when I told him that I was surviving everything else that was being thrown at me, so why not give me my chemo today anyway, I would probably survive it. But he was adamant - it was too dangerous. Home I went again, chemo-less.

Chapter 12

Losing my hair, losing my faith

I have now settled into a routine. Between visits for chemo and blood transfusions, the clinic has become like a second home. I know all the nurses, quite a few of the doctors and most of the Tuesday patients. It has become so familiar that I feel as if I spend as much time there as I do at home. I would rather not be there. What I really want is to be finished with the lot of it. But in addition to losing my hair, I am now losing faith in ever completing my chemo treatments.

Every Tuesday I arrive with the hope that I will get my chemo today, but mostly I am disappointed. Either my blood is misbehaving or I am not in good enough shape to have it. I now see Paul every time I visit the clinic. We have settled into a routine. We analyse my CA125 together then we move on to my blood - not that I know much about it, but he explains everything so that I understand. The blood results are usually bad - no chemo today. I have had a series of blood transfusions. They generally make me feel much better and I usually have more energy after them. I am beginning to see myself as a budding Dracula.

At home I am eating better and I now go for a walk with Vincey down to the bottom of the road and back a couple of times a week. It still exhausts me, but at least I am getting out. I sometimes bump into my neighbours and it is sad to see how embarrassed they are. They are not sure what to say to me. They can see that I look ill, but don't know whether to ask me what is wrong or not. I get around the problem by telling one of my closest neighbours what is happening and she says she will pass the word around. The reaction is almost miraculous. When I now see my neighbours they stop and ask me how I am and if I am making progress. All the embarrassment is gone.

The strands of my hair are falling out with the frequency of leaves off a tree in autumn. If this continues I will be bald by Christmas. I bought a wig before my chemo started, but I do not like it very much and so far have only worn it a couple of times. Rosemary had taken me to a shop in Paddington that specialised in wigs, but I could not find anything I really liked. Eventually I settled for one that was adequate. Years ago, in the Sixties, when I used to wear wigs because it was fashionable, I had a very good selection. But somehow it is different when you need to wear a wig.

Back at the clinic, the problems are continuing. My blood is misbehaving. Either my platelets are too low or my blood is refusing to clot. I have always seen myself as a pretty average sort of person. I don't generally get too upset and I try to live as reasonably calm an existence as possible. I wish I could say the same about my body.

I have never given any thought as to how I would react to a major illness. I don't think I ever expected to have one. I assumed that if I were unlucky enough to catch something really serious, I would behave in a normal way, just the same as everyone else. How wrong I was. To start with, there is no such thing as normal. Everyone is different and will behave differently. And secondly, while my exterior might be calm, there is nothing calm about the inside of my body. It is a raging wild thing that ignores every plea for normal behaviour and will behave in a totally unruly way at the drop of a hat. My blood misbehaving has become the norm. It refuses to clot and I can't get my platelets off the floor.

Whenever my blood refuses to clot, the nurses tell me to stay away from sharp instruments in case I cut myself and to be careful when walking in case I trip over. If by some mishap, I should cut myself and start to bleed, I am instructed to get myself to casualty immediately. There I will be given an injection to clot my blood and stop me bleeding to death.

My blood's aversion to clotting is causing me problems elsewhere. At home I am not allowed anywhere near the knife drawer and if I use anything but the bluntest knife in the house to eat with, it is confiscated. Vincey is like a mother hen, watching my every move.

The times I miss my chemo because my blood is misbehaving are becoming legendary. I am getting further and further behind with my treatment. It is now such a regular occurrence that I am surprised when I do have treatment. If it is not my blood refusing to clot, then it is my platelets that are too low. It is always something. At one stage, my bone marrow - the part of your body that produces the cells - went on a go-slow because it was fed up with being beaten-up by the chemo. I am losing faith in ever completing all of my chemo treatments.

With so much time spent in the clinic just sitting around waiting for my blood results, I have taken up a new hobby - people watching. I now know most of the women spread over the three-week cycle, mainly because I am there nearly every week. It is interesting to see their different reactions to the chemo. The lesson you learn is that no two people are the same.

Some of the women are very subdued and don't want to talk to anyone. They close off the space around their armchair by burying their heads in pillows and pretending to be asleep. Others cannot stop talking. They want to discuss every detail of their treatment, how they feel and how they are coping. It is understandable. While others bury themselves in books or newspapers.

Women hate losing their hair. It makes them feel unattractive. There is probably some deep psychological reason for this that I cannot explain. But there is no doubt it is one of the horrors of chemotherapy. I know I keep harping on about hair, but it is the second most important factor for the majority of women, after their treatment.

The loss of their hair tells them daily that they are cancer victims on chemotherapy. And while they all accept the necessity of chemo - they would probably not be alive without it - they wish that they did not have to lose their hair as well. Having the chemo is just about bearable, losing their hair piles on the agony.

The other thing that happens to you is that you learn a new language, a silent language, one that consists of what is not said. You ask a nurse a question in all innocence, and the reply is so vague that you are left wondering if this is some sort of code and you have to try to decipher it. It makes these types of conversations scary.

Part of the reason for this is that the doctor is the only person who can tell you about your condition. This makes sense, but it is scary for the timid and the shy that are reluctant to ask doctors any questions. They feel more comfortable with the nurses or the volunteers who puff up their pillows and bring them cups of tea and coffee as the chemo is fed into their arms. They become attached to them and find it easier to discuss their worries with them rather than a more formal approach with a doctor.

Yet the doctors are wonderfully approachable. The biggest problem they have is a lack of time. The clinics are packed to the gills, but despite this, they try to give as much time as possible to everyone, sometimes working long days without breaks.

My reaction to the doctors had changed. I was now deeply suspicious of everything they said and did, and if for any reason there was even the smallest change in my treatment, I wanted to know chapter and verse immediately. I knew that the doctors were my best chance of recovery, even if only for a short time, but I questioned everything they said.

As a test to find out if I was being told the truth, I would ask a doctor one question and then try out the same question on another doctor to see if the answer was the same. All this proved was that medicine is not an exact science. Doctors can only give you guidelines. Yes, they hope you will be cured, but there are no guarantees. No two people will respond in the same way to treatment. They will explain the situation as they see it, but the outcome could be different because people are different.

Today is a red-letter day for me. It is a Friday morning in late September and I have been out on my own for the first time since before I had the operation. I am so excited. I went for a walk around the block and stopped off at the newsagent for a newspaper on the way back. Oh what a lovely feeling to be able to do something so normal. I had been down to Barnes village a couple of times with Rosemary, but this was my first solo outing and I was like a child let loose in a candy shop. It took me about thirty minutes and when I returned I was exhausted, but exhilarated. My stomach still hurts when I walk any distance, but I can tolerate the pain if I am going to have successes like this. All of the time I was away, Vincey was on tenterhooks, hoping that there were going to be no problems. He had visions of me collapsing en-route and ending up in hospital. He looked so relieved when he opened the door to me and saw that I was still intact.

I continue to see Paul regularly at the clinic, mainly because I am missing so many of my chemo treatments. I need to turn up every Tuesday morning, hoping that I will get my treatment today. The rejection rate is now so frequent that the nurses just take my blood for testing rather than prepare me for chemo. I had started out with six appointments, but now I have lost count as to how many times I have been there.

It is about this time that Jean, my nurse, tells me that she will be leaving soon as she wants to do research and clinical trials. I know I will miss her.

She has become part of my Tuesday life, as well as my blood transfusions. I think I am proving to be one of her longest standing patients, but she is far too diplomatic to say so. But she tells me that she will still be around the hospital and I will see her in the chemo room from time to time.

I had now completed about four of my treatments. I am eating regularly and I am able to go for longer walks than previously. The reduced chemo is making me feel better, but I am wondering if it is having any impact on the cancer. My hair is getting thinner and thinner and I still have that awful white pallor. And my stomach, which is now my major problem, is still very sore and does not seem to be healing. I can only walk slowly.

Yet despite all these setbacks, I have reason for optimism. I did not get those awful blisters in my mouth that many women suffer from as part of their treatment. I had seen them in the clinic, sucking ice cubes to reduce the pain. I had been dreading the thought of them and used to drag myself out of bed to clean my teeth and wash my mouth out with a medicinal solution to prevent even the smallest infection. My feet are still numb, although they are not as sore, this could well be a permanent state. The chemo, apparently, can sometimes kill off the nerve endings in your toes and they cannot be repaired. My hands still have the red rash that is another give-away that you are on chemo. But when I take everything into consideration, I feel that I am making a slow, but steady recovery.

I must be improving. For the first time I went shopping in the supermarket close to where I live on my own. This is another red-letter day. But the shine is taken off the achievement because my hair is now so thin that I am wearing a hat. I walk up and down the aisles picking up what I want as I go along. The basket weighs a ton, yet there are only a couple of items in it. For some reason that I cannot explain, I feel really nervous. I think it is because I am scared that I am going to faint, but I get home with my shopping without mishap.

Next week, Rosemary and I are planing a trip to Hammersmith, using public transport. I know it is only one stop on the bus, but it will be another first, something that I have not done for months.

On Tuesday I meet my new nurse. Her name is Sue and she is from New Zealand. She is lovely and we hit it off immediately. The first thing I discover about Sue is that she is passionate about rugby, but she has a conflict of interest problem. She is the loyal supporter of two countries, which can cause her difficulties when they are playing each other and she has to try to support both simultaneously. As a New Zealander, she is fanatical in her support for the All Blacks. But she also supports Wales, the country of her mother's birth. When I meet her for the first time, she has no voice. I assume she has a cold and ask her what she is taking for it. With a self-conscious grin on her face, she tells me that she went to a rugby match in Wales at the weekend and her lack of voice is the result of over-enthusiastic cheering.

Later, I see Paul. We are looking at the latest results of my CA125. According to the screen, it is down to fifty, almost unbelievable at this stage. I voice my suspicions and Paul agrees with me. The leap down had been too big. We'll have to wait for the next test to see what the true numbers are. But the good news is that I am to have my chemo today. This is my fifth. I feel like shouting from the rooftops. Only one more left. At this rate I might make it to Madrid for Christmas. It is the one thing that has been driving me forward. Both Vincey and I can't wait to see our daughter, son-in-law and grandchildren again. It is nearly four months since we have seen them, the longest period ever. In the past, we went to Madrid about every two months. In between those times, Jackie would bring the children to London.

On Friday morning Rosemary and I set out for Hammersmith. Somehow, I seem to have less energy that usual and I take ages to walk down the road. By the time I reach the bottom I feel slightly fatigued, but I am determined. It is only one bus stop away, albeit a longish one over Hammersmith Bridge. I struggle on to the bus - the steps are proving too high and it hurts my stomach. Rosemary is all for going back home. She thinks that I am overdoing it. Although the bus is fairly full, a woman jumps up to give me her seat. I accept gratefully, but think to myself that I must be looking pretty awful.

We are only out for about thirty minutes when we have to return. I am in agony with pains in both my stomach and my back. We try to get a taxi, but a bus comes along first and we get on. I don't know when my next trip out will be. If I am like this going to Hammersmith, I am unlikely to make it to Heathrow never mind Madrid. All my new-found excitement at the though of leading a normal life again is evaporating into thin air.

When I next visit the clinic I tell Paul about the pains in my back, but particularly about my stomach, which is the worse of the two. He decides to send me for a scan to see if there is any reason for concern. I also ask him if we can have a review of my progress, which if you think about it is a bit silly. It is just that I seem to have been visiting this clinic forever and it would be nice to know that there is an end in sight. It proved to be the shortest and briefest review that I have ever known. Sitting there, I drew two sections on my pad - I take notes all the time now - all ready for a detailed listing of everything. To make sure that there were no misunderstandings, I drew a line down the centre of the page, marking one side positive the other negative. On the negative side, Paul says, "put down we nearly killed you." On the positive side, he says, "put down that we are curing you." When I asked him if that was it, he said, yes, that's it. But there must be something else that can be said, I countered. But apparently not. That was it. We both ended up laughing.

Yesterday morning I was putting my hat on to go for a walk when I noticed in the mirror what looked like newly grown hair on my head about a centimetre long. I run my hand over it not willing to believe my eyes. But it is true. I am astonished. It is not my imagination. There really is hair there. I call Vincey. "Come and look at my hair", I shout excitedly, but he says that he cannot see it.

He admits that he can feel some short hair, but that's all. To me, it is wonderful. My hair is growing back. Although I still have some of my existing hair, it is very thin. But this means that I was not going to be bald. I found the hair growth surprising because I had been told that the hair does not start to grow again until after the chemo is finished. Yet here it was in all its glory. When I saw Rosemary the next day I could barely contain myself. She was hardly in the front door before I was showing her my head and asking for confirmation that hair was really growing.

You acquire some strange habits after a major illness. Mine was about women wearing hats and scarves. I could not stop looking at them, sometimes to the point of rudeness. I had to know why they were wearing them. I was assessing them to see if I could work out whether the head covering was disguising the fact that they were having chemotherapy or they just liked headgear. It's not such a difficult task. Those hiding a lack of hair usually wear a particular type of hat – invariably the woolly pull on type. Others prefer a scarf tied turban-style round their heads. But the one thing that they all have in common is the need to cover up the hairline – that way you don't know whether they have hair or not. But you can assume that if their head is completed covered, they are having chemo.

Three weeks later I am back at the clinic and Paul has the results of my scan. He says that they cannot see anything wrong with my stomach or lungs and the reason I am in pain is probably because I am still sore from the operation. He then tells me that I should make an appointment to see Professor Gabra over at Queen Charlotte's. The professor is the head of both Hammersmith and Queen Charlotte's. I make an appointment for two weeks' time.

I don't get my chemo. My platelets are in very poor shape.

Chapter 13

At last, final chemo

On my final chemo, I tell myself, I will know whether all the months of misery and suffering will have been worth while. I will know whether the treatment has been successful or not. There was the possibility that despite my dogged perservance it had all been a complete waste of time and I was still riddled with cancer.

Now is the moment of truth. I will know good or bad. Today is the day that I had longed for all those months ago, craved, even dreamt about. It was going to be my eldorado. But it is proving to be something of an anti-climax. This is not how it was supposed to be. I should be feeling excited, anticipating good news. This was supposed to be the day when everything would be revealed. The day when I would know if I were going to live or die. I remember when I was on my second bout of chemo, I dearly wished that I was at this point - my final treatment. At the time, I could not envisage many more days or weeks like the ones I was experiencing – hardly able to move and with one day much the same as the next as they merged into each other. Now I was at the end of that long journey, a journey that had taken me through some of the lowest moments of my life.

But I already knew the results - even before my final chemo. I had seen Professor Gabra at Queen Charlotte's the previous Monday. I had never met the professor before and I was not sure what to expect. As it turned out, he was of Asian extraction and had one of the broadest Scottish accents I have heard in an age. Add to this a straightforward way of presenting the facts, a big, friendly smile and here was a very approachable cancer guru. He sits me down beside his desk and consults the screen. "Your CA125 has been down for two consecutive tests, so you are in remission," he says. My immediate reaction is to jump up and kiss him, but I restrain myself. Instead I babble on about everything and nothing. I seem to be suffering from that other disease - logorrhoea, or as it is more commonly known verbal diarrhea. I open my mouth and rubbish pours out. I cannot stop myself. When he gets a word in, he tells me that his assessment is based on my CA125 readings, and warned that it also requires a CT scan to confirm that no cancer is evident.

I can't wait to get outside and ring Vincey. I know he is hoping for the best, but fearing the worst. I tell him I have to get it confirmed with a CT scan. We will then be one hundred per cent sure. I will get the results of my scan when I go to the clinic in two weeks' time for my final chemo. The entire family is threatening to descend on me and have a party to celebrate. But I manage to talk them out of that.

Now that I am getting a much-reduced chemo dosage, I have late appointments. I had arrived at my usual time - nine forty-five for my ten o'clock appointment and went and saw Sue straight away. She did my bloods and I went and sat out in the main reception area to wait for the results to come back from the laboratory. If my body were still protesting, I would not have my chemo today. It had being postponed so many times that I no longer gave it any thought.

The clinic is packed and as I sit there, my thoughts turn to more practical matters as I survey what is now a very familiar scene - ashen-faced women with covered heads all sitting and waiting patiently for their turn. They are probably all wondering what today will bring for them.

I have a fair idea of what today is going to bring for me. But first I need an all-clear scan result and I need my final chemo. My thoughts drift to the future, no matter how short it may prove to be. If I am free of the cancer, even if it is only for a short time, I won't have to journey almost every week to this clinic. I won't have to sit and wait to hear the results of how my body is behaving this week. I won't have to ask myself the question: will I get my chemo today, or will it be another rejection. Oh, the joy of getting back to some sort of normality. No matter how much I like and appreciate the doctors and nurses, I will not be unhappy if I never see them again - medically-speaking, that is.

But I chide myself for not being more positive today. This is what all those previous months were about. This is what the operation was about, the first two overdoses when I had almost wished that I were dead, despite wanting to live for my family. This is the culmination of all those months of agony, of my family's agony and how they willed me to live, despite the fact that their eyes were telling them I was close to death. No matter how ill I was, they never gave up hope and were there, encouraging me, willing me on.

Suddenly I hear Iain calling my name. I go through to his office. "Good news," he says, "the scan has come back clear and you are also going to have your chemo today." I feel like crying, not something I am in the habit of doing, but say thank you instead. Iain, the ever-practical Scot, also sounds a warning. "Remember it can come back," he says. I know this already, but I want to savour the moment - no more clinic visits for the foreseeable future. I thank him for all his help and care and wish him every success in his new job - he is off to a hospital in the city to concentrate more on research.

Now sitting attached to my chemo drip for what I hope will be the last time, my thoughts drift back in time. During the worst days of my illness, when I was still unaware of the dangers of ovarian cancer, my most fervent wish was that I would survive long enough to see my grandchildren grow up. My thoughts drifted in this direction when I was at my lowest ebb and I would end up in floods of tears. Now I had to accept that unless the pharmaceutical industry comes up with a miracle drug very soon, I won't be around for long enough.

My attitude to cancer now is very different from what it was. You don't fight cancer. What you are fighting for is to get your life back to some sort of normality whereby you can do everyday things like going to work, going shopping, going out with family or friends. But normality comes with an edge. Before, you assumed that barring a fatal accident, you would get in your three score years and ten. That, however, is an assumption that you can no longer make. You have cancer and while your body may be free of it for the moment, you don't know when it will return and that makes every day that you survive precious. You live for each day and if you make it through the seasons, that is a blessing.

All of this is totally the opposite of my attitude when I was diagnosed with bladder cancer and breast cancer. It never crossed my mind that I would not survive. So far as I was concerned, it was life as usual. When the bladder consultant told me I would probably die of something else, I took it at face value and not once did I think that it would be the cause of my death. I took a similar attitude to my breast cancer.

A favourite expression of the cancer consultant is: "You don't know you are cured until you die of something else."

Basically, you and your family live with the shadow of cancer always hanging over you every day for the rest of your life. It is a treacherous disease.

Chapter 14

Awareness is vital

You will know by now that ovarian cancer is deadly and hard to detect. You will know that early diagnosis - stage one - is your best chance of survival.

There is no simple or easy test to identify it. The symptoms are such ordinary everyday ones that most women dismiss them from their thoughts as of no consequence. When did backache, heartburn or mild tummy ache become so dangerous? When did they start to kill women?

Yet they do. At least one hundred women lose their lives to ovarian cancer every week because they are diagnosed too late. The unpalatable truth is that they don't know they have the cancer until they are past the stage where they could be helped.

And if there are any doubts about the danger of this cancer, look at the survival rates. They are dire. Of the women diagnosed at stage three, seventy-five per cent will be lucky if they are still alive two years later. It is not choosy about whom it strikes either. It can affect anyone. I was shocked to discover that girls as young as eleven have died from it. But the age group most at risk is over fifty and accounts for the biggest number of deaths.

Another piece of information I discovered while I was researching this most secret of cancers is the link between breast cancer and ovarian cancer. If you have had breast cancer, you are a potential candidate for ovarian cancer.

Basically what this means is that if you have had breast cancer, you should be extra vigilant and demand annual checks. But no one tells you this.

Many months after I started to recover and was able to attend Queen Mary's Hospital in Roehampton for my delayed annual mammogram, that was my first question - why was I not told. When I challenged the consultant John Cummins, he explained that I had the wrong type of cancer.

I was not convinced. This sounded like a variation of one of those lame British Rail excuses used to explain the lack of train services - signal failure, wrong snow on the line. But he surprised me by volunteering information about another of his patients who had the same breast cancer as me and now had ovarian cancer as well. His conclusion: more research is needed that will either prove or disprove the link between these two types of cancer. Or it could just be a very big coincidence.

But all the research in the world will have little or no impact unless women take responsibility for their own bodies. Knowledge is power and the only way to have that power is to be aware of your body and any changes affecting it, no matter how minor. I am not suggesting that everyone takes up DIY medicine - just be aware and respond.

There is a practical and sensible way to monitor your body for ovarian cancer and here it is:

If you experience any of the following over a continuous period, take action.

Suddenly occurring backache lasting over a couple of weeks.

Heartburn.

Stomach ache - no matter how mild and also lasting over a couple of weeks.

Vaginal bleeding

General feeling of not being well.

Bloated stomach.

It is necessary to experience at least three of the above. That however does not mean that you have ovarian cancer. It just means that you should see your GP and get checked out.

If you believe that there is cause for concern, make an immediate appointment to see your GP. Ask for a CA125 blood test. This is not a guaranteed method of detection, but it is a very good tumour marker. The only drawback is that it sometimes shows positive when there is no cancer present or, worse still, it misses the cancer altogether. If you are over fifty or menopausal, your doctor can do a simple test that will either confirm your worst fears - you have the beginnings of a tumour - or there is nothing to worry about.

The next step, if there is even the slightest doubt, is to get your GP to organise an appointment for a transvaginal ultrasound. This will almost certainly confirm whether you have ovarian cancer or not.

It is essential that once cancer has been confirmed, action be taken. Delay can be fatal. If you are diagnosed positive, it is important that you see a specialist in ovarian cancer. Under the care of a good multi-professional specialist team, your chances of survival will improve dramatically. They will be aware of the latest research, the newest drugs and most importantly, they will be used to treating women with ovarian cancer daily. This gives them a major edge over other specialists - for not only do they have the expertise, but also the experience.

Being in the know also helps. It is helpful to be aware of the treatment you are receiving and that it is the best currently available. A good source of information for this is the Internet. If you are not online at home or at work, consider signing up at home. You will be amazed at the amount of good, solid information available about ovarian cancer and its treatment.

For those with Internet access at home, there is the added advantage of the support groups. The majority of the sites are in the US, but they address the same fears and concerns that worry women all over the world about ovarian cancer. And best of all, the women are happy to discuss their treatments and their fears openly. A short email to any one of the sites will produce gold dust. It also gives you the opportunity to gain knowledge and to keep yourself informed about the latest treatment and drugs being used. After all, the United States is one of the top countries in the world for research and development into cancers.

What I have discovered in the past decade as I journeyed around the NHS with my cancers is that while doctors are very open and will answer any question that you put to them, they seldom volunteer information. Part of the reason for this is that medicine is not an exact science and people have a tendency to react differently to treatments, which makes it difficult for the doctor. But it also makes it particularly arduous for the patient to get a complete picture of what is wrong, what the treatment should be and the possible after effects. Unless you are a doctor yourself, how do you know what questions to ask? That is why the Internet is such a bonus.

When I was first diagnosed, I asked every woman I came into contact with if she knew anything about ovarian cancer. I had my daughter and sisters asking the same question. The vast majority of those questioned had heard of it, but were totally ignorant of the symptoms and how dangerous it was. It is for this reason that I want to use whatever time I have left to improve awareness among women and their families. Without a possible cure on the horizon, the key to survival is early detection.

There is little more that I can say - I have told you my story and I have told you how my lack of knowledge nearly killed me and may yet do so. But I am not dead yet and, for as long as I can, I plan to become involved in raising money to fund an awareness campaign - an early warning system for women.

I hope I have the time to get my Internet site on ovarian cancer up and running. You will know if I am successful - you will be able to find me at www.embraceus.com. Take a look now and then to see if I am still alive.

Chapter 15

It's back.

It's back. Everyone is devastated, numb with shock. They cannot comprehend why it has returned so quickly. Even the hospital is surprised. Vincey is walking around looking stunned - he cannot believe it. He keeps saying to me that it's not fair - "You went through so much the first time and now it is back again."

We are back on the same old treadmill. Everyone is being positive. "You got though the first time," is the general chorus. "You'll get through this as well." But we all know that second time around is much more difficult.

I had the results of my blood test last week and my CA125 is raised. I have seen Professor Gabra and I am now waiting for the results of the CT scan and the kidney test. The results will tell whether I have weeks or months left and if there is any credible treatment. The one piece of good news is that the professor has told me that he is not giving up on me.

This is not a chapter I was expecting to be writing. I though it would come a little later, after the book was published. That's what I was hoping for - but it is not to be.

I had completed the last chapter on such a high. But if I am honest with myself, I was probably being too optimistic, remembering my previous encounters with cancer and thinking I could squeeze out another few months. I knew the statistics. I was expecting too much thinking that I might have a year. Have time to be able to do things, like promote an awareness campaign.

Vincey and I had promised ourselves that we would do a little travelling. Nothing too arduous or distant. He even volunteered to go to New York. Jackie wanted us to go and live in Madrid for a while so that we could spend more time with our wonderful grandchildren. I was considering it - even if it were only for a few months.

I am now fed up with cancer and what it is doing to my family and me. When it is over, I think it will be for the best. My poor, long suffering family might get a respite from my cancers and me. They deserve it. I may have had the cancers, but they endure every agonising step I take in trying to survive. And they do it without complaint and almost superhuman support, no matter how bad things become. They were there for me. What more could I ask for?

Chapter 16

Vincey

If I thought Chapter 15 was devastating, I hardly know how to describe Chapter 16.

Added at the last minute, just before printing, it is the worst one I have every written - tragedy beyond anything else that has happened to me. But this book could not have been published without it.

My Vince, my love has left me and I am consumed with grief. I can think of nothing else. He didn't want to leave me, but was taken by a heart attack, something that was always a possibility, but never expected.

My life is now a bleak hole, left empty by a man who loved me, cared for me, kept me alive during the worst moments of my illness when I would have been happy to die.

Now I am without him and all I can think of is how I can be with him. If tears could bring him back, he would be by my side now.

When you have stage three ovarian cancer, your survival rates are not good - probably a couple of years.

My two years are up in May and I am hoping that I will join him. I know this is selfish - I should think of my family, particularly my daughter and grandchildren, but all I can think of is Vincey and how soon I can be with him.

I am dedicating this book to Vincey - without him I would not have survived to write it.

OVACOME

The signs and symptoms of ovarian cancer

Ovarian cancer affects 7000 women in the UK each year. In the majority of cases the cancer has already spread by the time it is found. Ovarian cancer has the sinister reputation of being a silent killer. Why? Well it's mostly because of where the ovaries are- hidden deep inside the pelvis.

Most ovarian cancers start on the surface of the ovary. There are many different kinds of cancer. Some grow and spread rapidly, whilst others thankfully stay confined to the ovary. Women rarely have any symptoms at this early stage (stage 1), only noticing changes when the cancer gets larger, or when it starts to affect other organs.

Below is a list of signs and symptoms which many women have reported. Its important to realise that they are all pretty common. Having some of them does not mean you have cancer, but you should nonetheless get them checked out. Some women with ovarian cancer have no symptoms, and rather say that they 'just didn't feel right'. If you have concerns, then the most important thing is to talk with your GP.

Some of the signs and symptoms of ovarian cancer are:

Abdominal distension- some women reported that they looked pregnant, others that they felt bloated and full all the time.
Abdominal pain - many women have been treated for Irritable bowel syndrome
Indigestion or feeling sick
Urinary problems-needing to empty the bladder urgently
Change in bowel habit
Pain during sexual intercourse.

Most women have some of these symptoms at some point during their lives. Research in the USA by Barbara Goff shows that women with ovarian cancer have these symptoms, but they are more severe than women who have the symptoms due to another cause.

In the future, there will be screening methods to detect ovarian cancer at its earliest stage. There is currently a large study testing 2 screening methods, Ultrasound, and a blood test CA125. It is hoped that this trail will prove the reliability of these tests, and in the future, women in the UK will be diagnosed before signs and symptoms occur.

Women concerned about ovarian cancer can speak to trained nurses, with a special interest in ovarian cancer by contacting Ovacome. Ovacome is the UK support and information charity for those affected by ovarian cancer. Their support line number is 0207 380 9589.

OVARIAN CANCER ACTION

The UK has amongst the worst survival rates for ovarian cancer in the developed world. That's a hard fact to swallow. Of the 7,000 women diagnosed in this country each year, just 3 in 10 women are likely to survive five years or more in this country, compared to just over 5 in 10 in the United States. Unlike other cancers, there have been no significant developments in survival rates for well over 20 years.

Why do so many women die? Treatments are relatively standard around the world. The answer lies in the fact that most (75%) women are not diagnosed with ovarian cancer until it has already spread. Caught early, the survival rates are much, much higher.

Ovarian cancer action exists because it is determined to change those figures. We are committed to funding world class research in the UK, raising awareness of the signs and symptoms, and working with women to have their voices heard at the highest level.

We are the only national, single issue charity raising awareness, proactively, through national media campaigns and leaflets. In 2005 we reached over 37 million readers of magazines and papers in Ovarian Cancer Awareness Month. We're prepared to shout about the fact that this is NOT a silent killer. Yes it sometimes whispers, and GP's rarely see a case, but it is still the fourth most common cancer in women, and patients often spend months reporting symptoms before a correct diagnosis is made. Reliable screening tests, suitable for widespread use, and early diagnostic markers are realistically years away. Until that point, and arguably beyond, awareness will play a vital part, in getting women to their doctors as early as possible

Symptoms can include
- A constantly swollen abdomen
- Increased urinary urgency
- Feeling full or bloated
- Unexplained abdominal or back pain
- Changes in bowel patterns
- Ongoing excessive fatigue
- Onset of unexplainable indigestion or nausa
- Abnormal vaginal bleeding

Remember the cause is most likely something far less serious (such as irritable bowel syndrome or a benign cyst). However, if you develop a number of symptoms, that start suddenly for no reason, are very frequent and persistent, or you are being treated unsuccessfully for other conditions, please do talk with your doctor. You should also let your doctor know if 2 or more of your close relatives from the same side of the family, have had either ovarian or breast cancer, as around 1 in 10 cases have a genetic link. For full details of risk factors and symptoms, please visit our website www.ovarian.org.uk

All our work is carried out as a result of donations, legacies and corporate partnerships. If you would like to help us achieve our aims, please contact us either via the website at www.ovarian.org.uk by email info@ovarian.org.uk or by phone 020 8238 7605.